Living
with PCOS

Polycystic Ovary Syndrome

Second Edition

Angela Boss • Evelina Sterling
with Jerald S. Goldstein, M.D.

Addicus Books
Omaha, Nebraska

An Addicus Nonfiction Book

Second Edition
ISBN 978-10-886039-01-8
Cover design by Peri Poloni-Gabriel
Illustrations by Jack Kusler
Typography by Linda Dageforde

This book is not intended to be a substitute for a physician, nor do the authors intend to give advice contrary to that of an attending physician.

Library of Congress Cataloging-in-Publication Data
Best Boss, Angela
    Living with PCOS : polycystic ovary syndrome / Angela Best Boss and Evelina Weidman Sterling — 2nd ed. / with Jerald S. Goldstein.
        p. Cm.
    "An Addicus nonfiction book."
    Includes bibliographical references and index.
    ISBN 978-10-886039-01-8 (alk. paper)
1. Polycystic ovary syndrome. 2. Polycystic ovary syndrome.—Treatment. I. Sterling, Evelina Weidman, 1970- II. Goldstein, Jerald S., 1965- III. Title.
RG480.S7B47 2009
618.1'1—dc22   2009027922

Addicus Books, Inc.
P.O. Box 45327
Omaha, Nebraska 68145
www.AddicusBooks.com

Printed in the United States of America
10 9 8 7 6 5 4 3 2 1

Contents

iii

Foreword

Polycystic ovary syndrome (PCOS) may well be the most common endocrine disorder affecting women of reproductive age. For some women, the disorder is very easy to identify, with the classic signs of irregular menses, increased facial hair growth, and infertility; however, for others the signs are more subtle, making diagnosis difficult.

The underlying disorder of PCOS is a problem with the way your body handles insulin. The result is a buildup of insulin in the blood that causes a chain reaction in which your body produces increased levels of male hormones, which then inhibit ovulation and cause irregular menstrual periods. Difficulties with the body's ability to metabolize insulin also account for other manifestations of PCOS, including Type 2 diabetes, lipid abnormalities, and coronary artery disease. It is now recognized that PCOS involves both environmental and genetic components, and studies are ongoing to determine which specific genes are involved. However, it is likely that PCOS is attributable to multiple genes rather than to a single gene.

Given there are so many symptoms of this disorder, it is understandable that a gynecologist might focus on only one symptom, such as irregular periods, and treat the problem by prescribing birth control pills. A dermatologist may treat unwanted facial hair with laser therapy. However, it is important to look at the overall picture, because untreated PCOS can cause not only infertility and miscarriage, but also may lead to serious health problems, such as heart disease, diabetes, and endometrial cancer. Often, it is the patient who first realizes that her combined symptoms point to PCOS.

By understanding PCOS, you and your doctor can individualize treatment, depending on your goals. For example, if you are trying to regulate your cycles, birth control pills may be the best option. If you are trying to conceive, a different approach would be necessary, and still another type of treatment is called for if you are bothered by unwanted hair growth.

I hope you will find that this book provides information that enables you to ask doctors the right questions. By being knowledgeable and proactive, you will be able to seek the most current treatments available, and by managing your PCOS, you will greatly improve your overall health as well as ability to conceive.

Jerald S. Goldstein, M.D.

Introduction

For most women with PCOS, there comes a time when they say, "Ah-ha! So *that's* what I have!" That epiphany began for me one evening about twelve years ago, when I happened to watch a network television program about PCOS. I was diagnosed several months later. I have what is a typical case, having had many of the symptoms since puberty. I gained weight early on and had irregular menstrual cycles. As a young woman, I had pleasant older physicians who said that some women just didn't have periods and that I would probably have difficulty getting pregnant.

Surprisingly, getting pregnant with my daughter, Kaylyn, couldn't have been easier. Having a second child proved to be much more difficult. A few rounds of fertility medicines resulted in a second pregnancy, but an early miscarriage. Most recently, adding an insulin sensitizer has renewed my ovulatory cycles as well as my hope for another child.

This book is written out of a deep passion for women with PCOS, their families and friends, and the medical professionals who treat them. For years, trying to find accurate information about PCOS has been difficult at best. We, the authors, have both been diagnosed with PCOS and wanted the best, most up-to-date information available about the disease and its treatment so that we could make informed medical choices.

Throughout the book, a number of wonderfully strong and courageous women share their stories. We are grateful for their honesty. Their wisdom, insight, and experiences are equally as important. These women are powerful reminders that as lonely as this journey can sometimes feel, many have walked before us.

Although living with PCOS is not easy, we now have access to a wider range of treatments than ever before. Additionally, with the growth of support groups and Internet-based news sites and bulletin boards, there are thousands of women willing to walk with you. You are not alone.

Angela Best Boss

Ever since I was a teenager, I had always thought I had some kind of hormonal problem. When I told my doctor about my concerns, he told me to relax and my body would straighten itself out eventually. After that, I really didn't think about it too much until I wanted to have a baby.

My body never did straighten itself out. My symptoms only got worse. Since I had suspected all along that my hormones were not functioning properly, I made an appointment with an endocrinologist. Fortunately, he was very knowledgeable and immediately diagnosed me with PCOS. With the help of a fertility drug, *Clomid*, I was able to become pregnant twice and give birth to two beautiful children. I am just now coming to terms with my PCOS and how it affects my life. I continue to work with my doctors on an effective treatment plan that will hopefully help me live a long and healthy life.

Evelina Weidman Sterling

1

PCOS—A Complex Hormone Disorder

As soon as Debbie hit puberty, her periods became irregular. She gained weight faster than any of her girlfriends, and she was embarrassed by the amount of hair on her chin, arms, and legs. Her mother took her to their family doctor, who brushed off the symptoms, explaining that it would take a while for her hormones to "adjust."

Debbie is now twenty-eight, happily married, and ready to start a family. Unfortunately, she is still having the same problems. Her hormones still haven't "adjusted." As a matter of fact, it has been six months since her last period. When she talked to her doctor about this during her last visit, he indicated that she may be under too much stress and that she is a few pounds overweight. The doctor said tests weren't necessary; it was nothing serious. He said Debbie should just go home and relax.

However, Debbie cannot relax. She is frustrated and confused. She knows something is wrong, but what?

What Is PCOS?

Polycystic ovary syndrome, or *PCOS,* is a complex hormone disorder, characterized by an increased production of androgens (male hormones) and ovulatory dysfunction. It causes symptoms such as irregular menstrual cycles, infertility, excessive body hair (hirsutism), acne, and obesity. The syndrome is named for the cysts that may form in the ovaries when the hormone imbalance interrupts the ovulation process. The term *polycystic* means "composed of many cysts." If PCOS is left untreated, and the hormone imbalance continues, the syndrome can eventually lead to serious illnesses such as diabetes, heart disease, stroke, and endometrial cancers.

Symptoms of PCOS

Symptoms of PCOS usually begin to appear around the time a young woman starts having her menstrual cycle. However, symptoms can also appear for the first time when a woman is older, especially if she has gained weight. Because it is a syndrome, PCOS includes a set of symptoms. Women with PCOS can suffer from any combination of these symptoms. Some women may experience only one of the symptoms, while other women experience all of them. The severity of PCOS symptoms can vary widely from woman to woman. Talk to your physician if you suffer from one or more of these symptoms:

- Chronically irregular menstrual cycles or absent periods
- Infertility or difficulty conceiving (due to not ovulating)
- Type 2 diabetes or insulin resistance
- Obesity (more than 20 percent over ideal weight)
- Sudden, unexplained weight gain (even if you are still at normal weight)
- Adult acne
- Excessive hair growth (especially, dark hair on the face, chest, or abdomen)
- Male-pattern hair loss or thinning hair

It is possible to have these symptoms and not have PCOS. However, most women with these symptoms, especially irregular menstrual cycles, do have PCOS. In fact, 80 percent of women with six or fewer periods per year have PCOS.

Researchers have found some variations in the symptoms among different races. For example, while excessive body hair is found among 70 percent of American women with PCOS, it occurs only in about 10 to 20 percent of Asian women. Unfortunately, there is not enough evidence to explain why these variations in symptoms occur.

Female Reproduction System

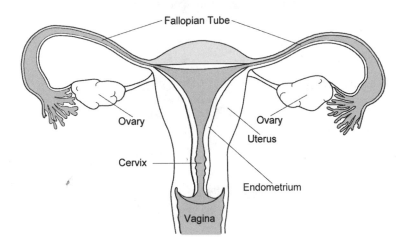

Worldwide Effort to Define PCOS

Because the symptoms of PCOS can vary widely, it can be difficult to exclude or include symptoms as a part of the diagnosis. In fact, the World Health Organization tried to determine a comprehensive list of symptoms and couldn't agree on more than four of them.

In 2003, a consortium of doctors from the United States and Europe gathered in Rotterdam to reach a consensus about PCOS symptoms. The intention of the Rotterdam PCOS consensus workshop group was to revise the guidelines that had been released by the National Institutes of Health in 1990. The Rotterdam panel determined that to be diagnosed with PCOS, a woman needed to meet two of three criteria:

- Irregular or absent ovulation (less than eight periods per year)
- Elevated levels of androgenic (male) hormones
- At least one ovary with twelve or more follicles or an enlarged ovary, greater than 10 millimeters in volume

The Rotterdam panel also determined that other factors could influence the diagnosis of PCOS. This included women who have regular periods but have polycystic ovaries on ultrasound and who have elevated androgens. A woman with PCOS would also have irregular menses and polycystic ovaries but no evidence of elevated androgens.

What Causes PCOS?

PCOS is the result of a hormonal imbalance, caused by a disorder in a woman's endocrine system. This system is made up of all the body's glands—pituitary, pineal, thyroid, parathyroid, thymus, adrenal, and pancreas. Hormones secreted by these glands control such things as growth, metabolism, and reproduction. In women with PCOS, this system is not working properly. Scientists believe there are several potential causes of this hormonal imbalance.

Insulin Resistance

Insulin resistance refers to the body's cells not responding to insulin, making it difficult to metabolize sugars. In other words, the body is resisting its own insulin. The hormone insulin is produced by the pancreas. Let's take a closer look at how insulin resistance occurs, starting with the intake of food. As food enters your body, it is broken down into small components, including *glucose*, an important sugar that comes from carbohydrates. Glucose is a major source of quick energy for the body. When you eat foods high in carbohydrates, your body detects a rise in glucose and signals the pancreas to produce more insulin.

Together, glucose and insulin enter the bloodstream. The insulin fits into special "insulin receptors" in the cells. This allows the excess glucose to enter the cells and to be converted to *glycogen*, which is then stored in the muscles and liver to be used later for energy. To use an analogy, think of insulin as the key that unlocks the body's cell door so that excess glucose can enter. When one has insulin resistance, it is as if the key no longer fits the lock. Consequently, the insulin is not able to fit into the insulin receptors, and excess glucose is not allowed to enter the cells. This causes a rise in both glucose and insulin levels in the blood.

For many years, PCOS was considered a direct result of high levels of male hormones in the body, although it was not understood exactly what caused these high levels. Researchers now understand the association between PCOS and the body's overproduction of insulin. An increase in insulin can stimulate androgen production. Subsequently, the body produces more male hormones and inhibits the ovaries

---

Symptoms of Type 2 Diabetes

- Fatigue
- Increased thirst and frequent urination
- Increased hunger
- Weight loss
- Blurred vision
- Slow-healing sores or frequent infections

---

from ovulating. This, in turn, causes the many PCOS-related symptoms.

Although insulin resistance is not found in every woman with PCOS, it is seen in many, most prominently in those who are overweight. If left untreated, insulin resistance can lead to Type 2 diabetes, defined as a condition in which the body either makes too little insulin or cannot properly use the insulin it makes to convert blood glucose to energy. Type 2 diabetes may be controlled with diet, exercise, and weight loss, or may require oral medications and/or insulin injections.

Genetics

It is unlikely that a single gene is involved in causing PCOS. It is more likely that multiple genes are involved. Research is ongoing to determine the role genes play. However, much of the data is difficult to gather since many women from previous generations were probably never diagnosed so it's impossible to know if they had PCOS. For example, there may be some women in your family who had difficulty getting pregnant but were eventually able to do so. Consequently, they may not think they had a problem with fertility. In addition, many of their other symptoms—hair growth and acne, for example—were either not serious or not important enough to mention to their physicians.

If you have a family history of adult-onset diabetes, infertility (or difficulty conceiving), obesity, or hirsutism (among women), then PCOS may run in your family. For example, if your sister has PCOS, there is a significant chance that you will also have PCOS.

Similarly, obesity can also increase the risk of developing the syndrome in those prone to developing it. Fatty tissues can produce estrogen, which can confuse the pituitary gland into secreting abnormal amounts of hormones, contributing to the overall endocrine problem. Some scientists speculate that women with PCOS are born with either a faulty gene or set of genes that triggers abnormally high levels of male hormones.

"There is no one officially diagnosed with PCOS in my family, but now that I have a better understanding of the condition, I see clearly that my mother has it and so did two of my dad's sisters and his mother. My dad is diabetic, as are several members of our extended family. No one takes me seriously when I try to get them to seek medical advice. They just count the diabetes and the heart conditions as the family curse," said Shelly, age twenty-nine, a woman with PCOS. "They don't consider that PCOS could be part of the culprit in our family's medical problems."

Researchers believe that the genetics of PCOS can also be passed on to males, who may experience some of the common symptoms. Male relatives of women with PCOS tend to be insulin resistant.

Who Gets PCOS?

The most common endocrine disorder, PCOS is estimated to affect anywhere from 5 to 10 percent of all women. At least 5 million and as many as 10 million women in the United States suffer from PCOS. It affects women of all ages, from adolescence to menopause. The syndrome does not discriminate and can be found in women of all races and ethnic groups throughout the world, although it tends to be more common in women of Mediterranean descent. Once a woman is diagnosed, she will need to manage the symptoms for the rest of her life.

Adolescent Females

Although the age of onset for PCOS symptoms varies, most women with PCOS can think back to their teenage years and remember a point in time when they started feeling "different" and wondering if something was wrong with them. Adolescent girls experience many of the same symptoms as adults—irregular or absent periods, unwanted hair, and acne. For many adolescents, these physical changes seem to occur

History of PCOS

This syndrome has baffled physicians for more than a century. In 1905, American gynecologists Dr. Irving Stein and Dr. Michael Leventhal were the first to officially describe PCOS. They both noticed a group of women who were experiencing similar symptoms—lack of periods, abnormal hair growth, obesity, and ovary enlargement caused by cysts.

These doctors were the first to link the seemingly unrelated symptoms and give the disorder a name, "Stein-Leventhal syndrome." Later, the disorder was renamed polycystic ovary syndrome, due to the polycystic ovaries that are found in many women who suffer from PCOS.

almost overnight. These girls might start to suddenly notice more and more dark hair on their chin and upper lip, or maybe their face is beginning to break out despite efforts to control it. In fact, their acne may be more severe than that of their friends.

Although young girls with PCOS may gain weight, it is important to know that PCOS, in itself, does not cause weight gain. PCOS, however, does make it difficult for a young girl to lose weight even though she is exercising regularly and eating well.

Adolescence can be a very difficult and emotional time for anyone. But for girls with PCOS, it can be even more difficult. They often feel isolated and confused. At an age when appearance is so important to them, girls with PCOS lose self-confidence as many of the symptoms start appearing. For many girls this feeling of confusion is exacerbated because they have no one to talk to for information or encouragement regarding their symptoms. Girls often feel too embarrassed to seek help or even mention what is happening to them. Additionally, mothers, friends, or other close adults often don't understand what is happening either. It's important to find a knowledgeable physician who can perform appropriate hormone tests to determine whether a teen has PCOS.

Some of the newer research suggests that girls who begin to develop pubic hair early (usually before the age of eight), a condition known as *premature pubarche*, have many of the signs and symptoms of PCOS. These girls have both elevated insulin levels and elevated levels of *dehydroepiandrosterone sulfate (DHEAS)*, a hormone secreted by the adrenal glands. An elevated level of DHEA is normally one of the first biochemical signs of awakening of the reproductive glands—in this case, the adrenal glands—after the long period of childhood inactivity. Throughout the rest of puberty, these girls produce excess testosterone and develop irregular periods consistent with PCOS. Thus, premature pubarche may be an early form of PCOS.

Women of Reproductive Age

The reproductive years typically refer to the years between the late teens and the mid-forties. It is during this time that many women are trying to conceive. Generally, a woman with PCOS will begin to experience menstrual irregularities within three to four years

11

after her first period. After menstruation starts, a woman may have a few years of normal cycles until the symptoms of PCOS become evident. In some cases, women continue into their early twenties with normal cycles or no apparent PCOS symptoms before the symptoms begin.

Most women are diagnosed with PCOS during their twenties or thirties. Many women are not diagnosed until they seek medical treatment after being unable to get pregnant. Because PCOS is often diagnosed only after a woman has trouble conceiving, those women who are not trying to become pregnant often are not diagnosed. But PCOS is much more than a fertility issue. Women who are not trying to become pregnant will still benefit from treatment.

It is still unclear how PCOS changes as women age, especially as they enter their thirties and forties. For some women, PCOS-related symptoms improve significantly as they get older. For others, the symptoms only worsen with age. Scientific research has not yet determined how factors such as weight loss, previous treatment with fertility drugs, or previous pregnancies or miscarriages affect women with PCOS over the course of their lives.

Menopausal Women

Menopause is the time in a woman's life when her menstrual cycle ends. Menopause typically occurs around age 50; however, it can occur at different ages. Many women experience the beginning stages of menopause in their 40s while others may not experience it as late as the age of 60. Menopause that occurs before age 40 is referred to as premature menopause.

Symptoms of menopause include irregular periods, hot flashes, vaginal dryness, decline in sexual interest, mood changes, and night sweats. Menopause is usually determined after a woman has not had a period for one year or more. PCOS can go unnoticed in menopausal women since they have irregular periods and often go for long stretches of time without menstruating at all.

Many women with PCOS believe that, since they have irregular periods, they won't go through menopause. However, this is not the case. It is important for menopausal women to seek treatment for both PCOS and menopausal symptoms.

Many women will take hormone replacement therapy (HRT) to relieve menopausal symptoms and to decrease the risk of developing osteoporosis. Because menopause causes a significant decrease in estrogen, many physicians prescribe estrogen. It can be given as a pill, topical gel, or patch. Some women, especially those with an intact uterus, are also given progesterone in addition to the estrogen. This helps protect the uterine lining against potentially harmful tissue changes, which can lead to endometrial cancer. The progesterone usually causes bleeding, similar to normal menstruation.

Unfortunately, hormone replacement therapy also comes with risks. Official guidelines recommend that women take HRT only for relief of menopausal symp-

toms and then at the lowest dose possible for the
shortest period of time possible. Extended use of hormone therapy has been linked to a variety of significant health problems, including breast cancer, heart
attack and stroke. It is important to discuss both the
benefits and risks with your doctor before you decide
to start hormone replacement therapy. Also, make
sure your health-care provider is familiar with PCOS
and can help you select a treatment plan that will take
into consideration the specific problems associated
with PCOS.

Since many women are now living well past their
eighties, the time spent post-menopausal can be thirty
or more years. We know that women with PCOS are
already at higher risk for developing diabetes, cardiovascular disease, and endometrial cancer. Because
such risks only increase with age, treating PCOS during and after menopause can minimize the risk of
developing these illnesses.

2

Getting a Diagnosis

Twenty-five-year-old Nicole had read a short article about PCOS in a popular women's magazine. She seemed to have many of the symptoms—being overweight, having excess body hair, and experiencing irregular periods. She was sure she had PCOS. However, she had just moved to a new city three months earlier and did not have a gynecologist. And, she felt she would be embarrassed to discuss her symptoms and concerns with a doctor she didn't know.

One year later, she made an appointment with a doctor whom a friend had recommended. The doctor asked questions about her medical history and also explained that, although her symptoms indicated she could have PCOS, there was no way to confirm the diagnosis without some simple tests. Nicole agreed to have an ultrasound to determine whether her ovaries were enlarged and some blood tests to measure hormone levels.

A few days later, the doctor called Nicole to confirm that she had PCOS. Nicole was relieved to finally understand her problem. Together, she and the doctor discussed various treatment options. Now Nicole wishes she had seen a doctor sooner.

Why Diagnosis May Be Difficult

PCOS is greatly underdiagnosed. It's estimated that only about 10 percent of women with the syndrome have received a diagnosis. PCOS is often difficult to diagnose for several reasons. First, many women are embarrassed about their symptoms and do not report them to their physicians. Also, women often do not recognize that the various symptoms can be the result of a single cause.

Compounding the problem, many physicians lack current knowledge about diagnosing and treating PCOS. They may attribute PCOS to other causes, especially lifestyle factors such as too much stress or excess weight gain.

Choosing a Physician

Women with PCOS often complain that finding a good health-care provider who understands the disorder can be tough. Although many physicians are not knowledgeable about PCOS, the situation is improving. Physicians are becoming more familiar with this condition, and women with PCOS are becoming more informed and aggressive in their search for treatment.

Many women have seen several doctors before finding the right one. There are several ways to find a good physician to manage your PCOS. First of all, you can contact the Polycystic Ovarian Syndrome Association (PCOSA). This organization maintains a state-by-state listing of member physicians who are interested in treating women with PCOS. More information is available at www.pcosupport.org. Also, you can contact RESOLVE, an international support group for women experiencing infertility, for a listing of physicians in your area who specialize in infertility issues. Visit their Web site at www.resolve.org.

Other possible sources for finding a physician include your primary care provider, a hospital network's referral services, insurance companies, or other professional associations such as the American Society for Reproductive Medicine and the Endocrine Society. When selecting a physician, remember to take into consideration your health insurance plan and proximity to the physician's office. Managing PCOS is an ongoing process and may require many visits to your doctor's office.

When selecting a physician, consider asking the following questions:

- **How soon can an appointment be scheduled?** Most women with PCOS have already seen several doctors who have not provided them with a proper diagnosis for their symptoms. Therefore, many of these women are eager to see a knowledgeable physician and might find it difficult to wait several months for an appointment. Also, find out how long you will

have to wait to see the doctor again for follow-up care. Find out if your doctor will be
available for telephone consults if you have any
further questions about your diagnosis or treatment.

- **Is there a physician in the practice who
  specializes in PCOS?** Ask the physician how
  many women with PCOS he/she has treated
  and how he/she typically treats it. This will give
  you a good idea as to the physician's current
  experience in helping women overcome PCOS
  symptoms.

- **What is the physician's background?** Ask
  about education, experience, and years in practice. Being diagnosed with and treated for PCOS
  can be very emotional, so try to select a physician with whom you will feel comfortable.

- **How does the physician typically diagnose
  and treat PCOS?** A physician begins by taking
  a detailed medical history, including a menstrual
  history. This is followed by obtaining lab studies
  and possibly imaging studies such as a transvaginal ultrasound. Decide how you would like
  to progress in your treatment of PCOS. If you
  are trying to become pregnant, do you want to
  be aggressive or do you prefer to take it slow?
  Once you have made a decision, select a physician who will meet your expectations.

- **Does the physician typically test for insulin problems and prescribe insulin-sensitizing agents?** Research stresses the link between PCOS and insulin resistance. It is important to make sure that your physician is aware of this research and is incorporating this information in how he/she addresses PCOS.

- **Does the health-care provider integrate or recommend natural or dietary therapies?** Since not every therapy works for every woman, some women are looking for a more-holistic approach. More and more evidence is showing the importance of nutrition and exercise in managing PCOS. If this type of treatment interests you, make sure you select a physician who supports your views.

Most women first turn to their obstetrician/gynecologist (OB/GYN) or primary care physician when looking for a diagnosis. Some women with PCOS end up seeing several OB/GYNs before they find one with whom they feel comfortable. The key is to not give up.

Since many women see nurse practitioners, physician assistants, or certified nurse-midwives for gynecological care, these health-care providers are becoming more and more knowledgeable about PCOS and are often able to make an accurate diagnosis. However, they are often more limited than physicians in their ability to provide a wide range of treatments.

Many women with PCOS, especially those who are trying to become pregnant, decide to see a specialist called a *reproductive endocrinologist (RE)*. REs focus on women or couples who are having difficulty conceiving, including those with PCOS.

If you are not trying to get pregnant and still would like to see a specialist, you might want to try a *general endocrinologist*, a physician who specializes in all hormonal disorders, or a reproductive endocrinologist whose practice is not limited to infertility.

Since PCOS can encompass a wide range of symptoms, it is possible that you will see a number of different types of health-care providers. For example, you may see a cardiologist for your high cholesterol and a dermatologist for acne. These physicians may want to prescribe different medications that treat each symptom individually. Therefore, it is important to make all your health-care providers aware that you have PCOS and explain what medications you are taking. It will also be your responsibility, as the patient, to find health-care providers who will be aware of treating your PCOS completely and not each symptom individually.

Your Medical History

During your first appointment with the physician you've chosen, he or she will likely ask questions about your personal and family history to see how it relates to PCOS. You will probably be asked the following questions about your menstrual history:

- Age at first period
- Length of menstrual cycle
- Regularity of menstrual cycle
- How your periods have changed over time
- How much bleeding is present during a cycle
- Period-related symptoms—pain, bloating, headaches

In addition, you will be asked about your reproductive history:

- Birth control methods used in the past
- Length of time you have been trying to get pregnant
- Number of pregnancies
- Number of miscarriages and/or abortions
- Menstrual irregularities or infertility issues experienced by your mother, sisters, or aunts

While your physician is collecting this information, it's important that you are completely honest. You will also want to discuss in detail with your physician all the symptoms that you have been experiencing, even if you are embarrassed or don't think they relate to PCOS. Also, let your physician know if you have a family history of infertility, diabetes, heart disease, stroke, or cancer. Once a diagnosis is obtained, you and your physician can work together to decide on your treatment goals.

Diagnostic Testing

There is not one specific test that a doctor can perform to determine whether you have PCOS. Nor can a physician make a diagnosis based solely on reported symptoms. However, by taking symptoms and family history into consideration, a physician can diagnose PCOS through a series of diagnostic tests. These include blood tests, which measure blood sugar levels and hormone levels. Also, a transvaginal ultrasound can determine whether the ovaries are enlarged.

Blood Sugar Levels

As mentioned earlier, when you have insulin resistance your body is not metabolizing sugars adequately. Four outcomes are possible when your blood sugar levels are tested. You may have:

- *Normal levels:* Your blood sugar levels are in the normal range, indicating that your body's insulin is keeping sugar levels under control.
- *Impaired fasting glucose:* Blood sugar tests during fasting are above normal but not high enough to be classified as diabetes. This is a prediabetic state that may progress to Type 2 diabetes if not brought under control with diet and exercise.
- *Impaired glucose tolerance:* Blood sugar levels are above normal after drinking a sugar solution

during a glucose tolerance test, but do not yet meet the criteria for a diagnosis of diabetes.

• *Type 2 diabetes:* Blood sugar test results meet the criteria for diabetes.

There are two blood tests commonly used to check blood sugar levels. The first one is the *fasting plasma glucose (FPG) test,* a simple blood test taken after eight hours of fasting. This test is the one most commonly used to check blood sugars. It is designed to determine the normal, baseline amount of glucose in your blood on an average day. The American Diabetes Association considers it the screening test of choice for diagnosing diabetes.

Most medical experts have established 100 mg/dL or below as normal. If you have a fasting blood sugar level between 100 and 125, you are classified as having "impaired fasting glucose," and are at high risk for Type 2 diabetes, high blood pressure and high cholesterol. If your level is above 126, you are considered to have diabetes, according to the American Diabetes Association.

Fasting Blood Sugar Classifications

Normal: less than 100 mg/dL
Impaired fasting glucose: 100–125 mg/dL
Diabetes: greater than 126 mg/dL

The second blood test, the *glucose tolerance test (GTT)*, is more sophisticated. It includes a fasting plasma glucose test, along with blood tests, based on blood being drawn at several intervals over a period of two to three hours after you drink a glucose solution. Normally, blood sugar increases modestly after drinking the glucose beverage and decreases after two hours. In the person with insulin resistance, the initial increase is excessive and the level remains high.

Glucose Tolerance Test Classifications

Normal: less than 140 mg/dL
Impaired glucose tolerance: 140–199 mg/dL
Diabetes: greater than 200 mg/dL

Another blood test, the *hemoglobin A1c test* also referred to as "A1c" also evaluates blood sugar levels. This test calculates how blood sugar levels have acted over the last three to four months. Hemoglobin A1c is a blood protein in red blood cells that bonds with blood sugar. Since red blood cells can live from 90 to 120 days, the hemoglobin A1c stays in the blood for that length of time. Accordingly, it is effective in measuring blood sugar over a period of months. Most doctors routinely run this test every few months for people who have diabetes. A normal level is less than 6 percent hemoglobin A1c. Some doctors prefer an even lower 5.5 percent.

Testosterone Levels

All women have some amount of the male hormone testosterone in their bodies, but women with PCOS often have increased levels of testosterone. To determine the amounts of the hormone present, your doctor may measure your *total testosterone*, which is the total amount in your body. However, most of the total testosterone is bound up by other proteins in the blood and is not biologically active. Therefore the doctor may also measure your *free testosterone*, which is the amount of the hormone circulating in your body and available to the cells. Free testosterone significantly contributes to such symptoms as excessive hair growth, baldness, and acne.

Some women with PCOS have testosterone levels that are still within the "normal" range, although often on the high end of "normal." However, even a slight increase in testosterone in a woman's body (even if it is within the "normal" range) can suppress normal menstruation and ovulation and lead to other PCOS-related symptoms.

Testing testosterone levels also helps a doctor rule out the possibility of adrenal or ovarian tumors.

Luteinizing Hormone and Follicle-Stimulating Hormone Levels

Luteinizing hormones (LH) and *follicle-stimulating hormones (FSH)* are secreted by the pituitary gland in the brain. These hormones stimulate ovulation. At the beginning of the menstrual cycle, LH and FSH levels are usually about equal. However, roughly twenty-four hours before ovulation occurs, the amount of LH increases significantly. This surge in LH is what causes the egg to be released from the ovary. Once the egg is released by the ovary, the LH level goes back down to its original pre-surge level.

Many women with PCOS already have an elevated LH level, so the amounts of LH and FSH at the beginning of the cycle are no longer equal. Although some women with PCOS still have LH and FSH levels that appear within the "normal" range, their LH level is often two or three times or more than that of the FSH level. This situation is called an *elevated LH to FSH ratio*. Because the amounts of LH and FSH should be very similar, this change in the LH to FSH ratio is enough to disrupt ovulation.

DHEAS Levels

DHEAS (dehydroepiandrosterone sulfate) is another male hormone that is found in all women. It is secreted by the adrenal glands. Women with PCOS often have elevated DHEAS levels. Similar to the testosterone levels, DHEAS levels that appear within the higher limits of the "normal" range are common among PCOS women. However, depending on the individual, even a minor increase in DHEAS, especially in conjunction with an increase in testosterone, can contribute to PCOS-related symptoms.

Androstenedione Levels

Androstenedione is another male hormone that is produced by the ovaries and adrenal glands. Sometimes, high levels can affect estrogen and testosterone levels, which, in turn, can contribute to PCOS-related symptoms.

Prolactin Levels

Prolactin is the hormone that stimulates and sustains milk production in nursing mothers. Prolactin levels are usually normal in women with PCOS. However, some women with PCOS have a slightly elevated level of prolactin, or *hyperprolactinemia*, which tells the body to produce milk. It can sometimes cause a white discharge from the breasts, even if you are not pregnant. It is important to check for high prolactin levels in order to rule out other problems, such as a pituitary tumor, that might be causing symptoms similar to those caused by PCOS.

Also, elevated prolactin levels interfere with normal ovulation and cause a woman to have short periods of no periods at all.

Progesterone Levels

After ovulation occurs, the hormone *progesterone* is produced by the *corpus luteum*, a yellow-colored mass in the ovary formed when the ovarian follicle has matured and released its egg. This process helps to prepare the uterine lining for pregnancy. Testing levels of progesterone is especially important. Sometimes, women with PCOS can show signs that ovulation is occurring; however, when the progesterone test is done, it shows that ovulation did not occur. If this happens, your body is producing a follicle and preparing you to ovulate, but for some reason, the egg is not being released from the ovary.

In addition, low progesterone levels may tell your doctor that your body is not producing enough progesterone on its own to sustain a pregnancy even if the egg is being released. All this information can help your physician adjust fertility medications for the next cycle to encourage the release of the egg and help sustain a pregnancy.

Estrogen Levels

The female hormone *estrogen* is secreted mainly by the ovaries and in small quantities by the adrenal glands. The most active estrogen in the body is called *estradiol*. A sufficient amount of estrogen is needed to work with progesterone to promote menstruation. Most women with PCOS are surprised to find that their estrogen levels fall within the normal range. This may be due to the fact that the high levels of the male hormone androgen found in women with PCOS can sometimes be converted to estrogen.

Thyroid-Stimulating Hormone Levels

Thyroid-stimulating hormone (TSH) is a pituitary hormone and controls the thyroid gland. Women with PCOS usually have normal TSH levels. TSH is checked to rule out other problems, such as an underactive or

Hormone Value Classifications
Normal Range and PCOS Range

	Normal Range	PCOS Range
FSH	Cycle Day 3: 3–12 mIU/ml	Most often, FSH levels fall within the normal range. FSH and LH levels should be roughly equal at Cycle Day 3.
LH	Cycle Day 3: 5–20 mIU/ml; "Surge" Day: 25–40 mIU/ml	For Cycle Day 3, sometimes LH levels fall within the normal range; however, LH is often elevated, making it two or three times greater than the FSH level. For "Surge" Day, often women with PCOS are unable to detect a surge of LH during their cycle, meaning that they are not ovulating.
Estrogen or Estradiol	Cycle Day 3: 25–75 ng/ml	Should be within normal range
Progesterone	Cycle Day 21 (or 7 days post ovulation)	Greater than 3ng/ml
Prolactin	Less than 25 ng/ml	For most, should be within the normal range. For some, slightly elevated prolactin levels, falling within the 25–40 ng/ml range.
TSH	0.4-5.0 mIU/L	Should be within the normal range
Total Testosterone	6.0–86 ng/ml	Usually greater than 40 ng/ml
Free Testosterone	Less than 5 ng/ml	May be elevated
DHEAS	35–430 ug/dL	Usually greater than 350 ug/dL
Androstenedione	0.7–3.1 ng/ml	Usually elevated

overactive thyroid, which often causes irregular or absent periods and no ovulation.

Hormone Ranges Vary

It is important to remember that hormone levels among women can vary greatly, and the variations mean that women don't always have the same symptoms. It is also important to mention that the "normal" ranges can vary since each lab sets its own "normal" values. Some women with hormone levels that appear within the "normal" range still suffer from symptoms and still might have PCOS. This is especially true with testosterone, DHEAS, and LH levels. Even small changes in these hormone levels can cause PCOS symptoms.

The table of normal hormone values in this chapter is a tool you can use with your physician to discuss your hormone levels and what they mean. As mentioned earlier, the diagnosis of PCOS is not based on a single blood test. For example, you can have a normal glucose level and still have PCOS. A physician makes the diagnosis of PCOS by considering these hormone values as well as by collecting a detailed patient history; the doctor also wants to exclude other ailments that may be causing symptoms.

Cholesterol Levels

Your physician will likely check your cholesterol levels as part of the blood testing procedures. Research shows that women with PCOS have a greater

Cholesterol Classifications

Cholesterol	Classification
LDL Cholesterol (mg/dL)	Optimal: less than 100
	Near or above optimal: 100–129
	Borderline high: 130–159
	High: greater than 160-189
HDL Cholesterol (mg/dL)	Low: less than 40
	High: greater than 60
Triglycerides (mg/dL)	Desirable: less than 150
	Borderline high: 150-199
	High: 200-499
Total Cholesterol (mg/dL)	Desirable: less than 200
	Borderline high: 200–239
	High: greater than 240

tendency toward high cholesterol levels. Cholesterol is a lipid, which is a waxy, fatlike substance found in every cell. The body normally uses these lipids to form cell membranes and hormones. Cholesterol is carried throughout the body by blood. If high cholesterol levels are left unchecked, they contribute to *atherosclerosis*, which is a buildup of fatty deposits that can cause blockages in the arteries.

There are two types of lipoproteins: *low-density lipoproteins (LDL)* and *high-density lipoproteins (HDL)*. A third type of lipid, *triglycerides*, are also components of cholesterol.

LDL

The low-density lipoproteins (LDL), or so-called "bad" cholesterol, can mix with other substances, forming *plaque*, which builds up in artery walls and may cause dangerous blockages. The particle size of the LDL determines the degree of danger. For example, Pattern A, which is made up of larger and "fluffy" particles, is the least dangerous form. Pattern B is made up of small and dense, or concentrated, particles and is considered the most dangerous form because the particles are capable of easily entering the arteries and forming plaque. High LDL levels increase the risk of atherosclerosis, or hardening of the arteries, and stroke.

HDL

The high-density lipoproteins (HDL) are considered the "good" cholesterol. HDL acts as a scavenger as it travels through the bloodstream, eating away at harmful cholesterol and carrying it away from the arteries and into the liver for excretion from the body. This action prevents the formation of clogged arteries (atherosclerosis). When HDL levels are too low, this cholesterol is not able to do its job well.

Triglycerides

Another component of cholesterol, triglycerides tend to be high in women with PCOS, further contributing to the risk of heart disease. Triglycerides are stored in fat tissues. When the body needs energy, the adipose tissue breaks down the triglycerides and releases them into the bloodstream as fatty acids. In obese individuals, too much fatty acid is released, and

Normal Ovary

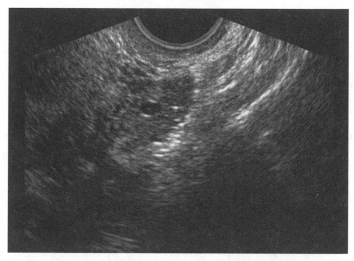

Cystic Ovary

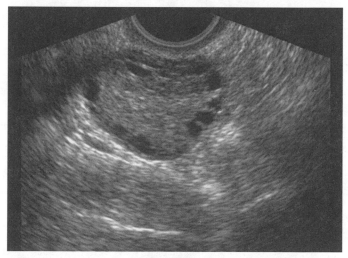

The top photo shows a normal ovary. The ovary shown in the bottom photo is from a woman with PCOS. Notice the enlarged follicles.

tissues become overloaded with fat, contributing to insulin resistance.

Triglycerides are also the most common form of fat in your diet. The majority of fats you eat, including vegetable oil and animal products, contain triglyceride molecules. Also, carbohydrates are converted to triglycerides by the body. When you eat more carbohydrates than you need, the body converts the excess calories to triglycerides, which are then stored as fat.

Examining the Ovaries

A tool for diagnosing enlarged ovaries, which are common in many women with PCOS, is the *transvaginal ultrasound.* This method uses sound waves to produce images of your reproductive organs on a video screen. In this procedure, the doctor inserts a handheld, cylinder-shaped instrument called a *transducer* into your vagina. Your doctor will move the transducer within your vagina to measure your ovaries to see if they are enlarged, to determine whether you have any cysts, and to view your *endometrium*—the lining of your uterus. For most women, the transvaginal ultrasound only takes a few minutes and is no more painful or uncomfortable than a regular pelvic exam.

Goals for Treatment

Once you've been diagnosed with PCOS, what are your goals for treatment? Each woman's personal goals vary when she is considering medical therapy for PCOS. For some women, bringing insulin to normal levels or getting pregnant may be the ultimate goal. For others, addressing cosmetic symptoms such as hirsutism may be high on the list. What matters most to you? Make a list of the main symptoms of PCOS that you wish to address. When you see a health-care provider, discuss these priorities.

3

Treatment of PCOS Symptoms

Rene, age twenty-nine, was delighted to begin treatment for PCOS. She had wanted to start a family, but PCOS had prevented her from ovulating regularly. Previous treatments, prescribed by other doctors, had been unsuccessful. Only after finding a new gynecologist did she feel hopeful. It had been just six months since she had started seeing the physician, who had been recommended by a woman in her PCOS support group. The new doctor was well informed about PCOS, had asked a lot of questions, and had listened to Rene explain her symptoms.

After beginning a new drug regimen, Rene's symptoms diminished. Although she wasn't pregnant yet, for the first time ever her menstrual cycles were normal. At last, Rene felt that a treatment was working.

Treating the Symptoms

There is no cure for PCOS, but with proper treatment, you can minimize the risk of future health problems. Several medications are used to treat women with PCOS who have insulin resistance and irregular menstrual cycles. Some of these drugs can have multiple benefits, improving several symptoms. However, there is no uniform pill or prescription for everyone. Women's symptoms vary, and they may respond differently to drugs. Accordingly, you and your physician need to work at finding the right drug or combination of drugs that alleviate your symptoms.

PCOS Symptom: Insulin Resistance

Insulin resistance was mentioned in previous chapters. As you'll recall, it occurs when the body does not allow its own insulin to carry glucose into the body cells, and sugars are not metabolized adequately.

Treatment for Insulin Resistance

Drugs known as *insulin sensitizers* are commonly prescribed for insulin resistance. Originally prescribed to people with Type 2 diabetes, these medications have also been shown to help women with PCOS who have insulin resistance. The sensitizers help the body recognize the insulin, allowing for the entry and storage of excess glucose in the body's cells. As insulin and glucose levels return to normal, many of the other hormones return to more-normal levels. In turn, many PCOS symptoms diminish. For many women, insulin sensitizers restore ovary function and menstrual cycles; often, the sensitizers alleviate such symptoms as excess body hair or thinning hair, acne, and excess weight. Insulin sensitizers also lower the risk of cardio-vascular disease and diabetes.

Serious side effects with insulin sensitizers are rare; however, they can cause liver problems, so your physician should monitor your liver function with periodic blood tests if any of these medications are prescribed for you. The insulin sensitizers most commonly prescribed for women with PCOS are *Glucophage, Fortamet, Actos, and Avandia.* These drugs have not been linked to liver problems. Still, if you are taking any of these medications, call your health-care provider right away if you develop nausea, vomiting, stomach pain, loss of energy or appetite, dark urine, or jaundice (yellow coloring of the eyes and skin). These may be symptoms of potential liver problems.

If you are taking insulin sensitizers, report any changes in your monthly cycle to your doctor. In addition, let your health-care provider know if you are trying to become pregnant, are already pregnant, or are breast-feeding. Insulin sensitizers are not approved by the FDA for use during pregnancy; however, many doctors consider them safe and prescribe them "off-label," meaning they've been approved for insulin resistance, but not approved for insulin resistance during pregnancy.

Metformin (Glucophage)

One insulin sensitizer used to treat PCOS is metformin. Approved by the FDA as a treatment for diabetes, metformin lowers insulin levels, and should be used in women who demonstrate glucose intolerance. The drug is sold under the brand names *Glucophage, Glucophage XR,* and *Fortamet.*

"I am so glad I decided to take it," said Julie, age thirty-eight. "Since being on metformin, my outlook on life in general has greatly improved. I am not tired all the time, and, most importantly, I enjoy playing with my kids again. I had a few gastro side effects—a little diarrhea and a little nausea. I even lost weight without changing my eating habits, although I am not sure if that has anything to do with the nausea."

Approximately 30 percent of patients started on Glucophage will experience gastrointestinal symptoms: diarrhea, nausea, vomiting, abdominal bloating, flatulence, and loss of appetite. These side effects are usually temporary (one to four weeks) and will disappear during continued therapy. It is advisable for new patients to initiate therapy slowly to minimize the gastrointestinal side effects.

"My endocrinologist said, 'Take this with food to avoid the GI upset.' I found I did best by taking the metformin halfway through the meal," Julie explained. "The food 'cushions' the pill, and the GI upset is lessened or in many cases eliminated. You may have diarrhea or nausea for approximately seven days minimally, regardless of what you do, so don't give up if that happens. Keep using it and you'll see a significant improvement."

According to some women, metformin's side effects may also include hair loss. This may prove too much for women already coping with thinning hair. The drug has also been associated with a rare condition called *lactic acidosis*, in which too much lactic acid, a by-product of carbohydrate metabolism, builds up in the bloodstream. This condition is potentially life-threatening. However, reported cases have occurred primarily in diabetic patients with severe renal (kidney) insufficiency.

Pioglitazone (Actos)

Another insulin sensitizer, *pioglitazone,* sold under the brand name *Actos,* ultimately normalizes other hormones, especially testosterone and LH. Another added benefit seen with pioglitazone is a reduction in the levels of triglycerides, fat-carrying molecules, which are one component of cholesterol.

Most people are able to take Actos with no problems; however, side effects are possible. They include upper respiratory infections, headache, muscle pain, sore throat, and swelling or fluid retention.

Rosiglitazone (Avandia)

The action of the drug *rosiglitazone,* whose brand name is *Avandia,* also improves insulin sensitivity. Avandia can be used alone or in combination with metformin. A low incidence of side effects was noted in clinical trials. Side effects of Avandia may include headache, backache, fatigue, and swelling or fluid retention. If you have heart failure, fluid retention, or active liver disease, your health-care provider will evaluate you to decide if Avandia is appropriate.

PCOS Symptom: Irregular Menstrual Cycles

If you have irregular periods, you have experienced the stress this causes. You may find yourself wondering whether you're pregnant, or you may worry about the embarrassment of starting your period when not prepared. Why does PCOS cause irregular cycles? It involves the balance of hormones. A woman's menstrual cycle is a perfectly synchronized process that occurs monthly. If a hormone level is abnormal, many other hormones are affected and the entire cycle is disrupted. This is what happens to women affected by PCOS.

Normally, a woman's body contains low levels of the male hormone androgen. However, in women with PCOS, these levels are elevated. Even a small elevation in the hormones testosterone and DHEAS can disrupt the menstrual cycle. They affect the feedback between the pituitary gland and the ovaries, leading to an abnormal production of LH and FSH—the hormones that stimulate the ovaries and promote ovulation. In women with PCOS, the level of LH is frequently, but not always, higher than usual, trying to start the cycle. As a result, the follicles containing eggs never develop, but instead turn into small, pea-sized cysts on the ovaries.

High levels of androgens also interfere with the FSH and LH that is needed to trigger progesterone, which controls the shedding of the uterine lining and menstruation. Surprisingly, despite all this, estrogen levels are generally normal in women with PCOS. This is due largely to the high levels of androgens, which are converted by the body into estrogen, keeping the estrogen level within the normal range.

PCOS-related menstrual irregularities can be a vicious cycle of *anovulation*, or not ovulating, and *amenorrhea*, or not menstruating. Although some women with PCOS stop having menstrual cycles altogether, other women continue having their cycles. However, their cycles are usually highly irregular. This irregularity is called *oligomenorrhea*.

Treatment for Irregular Menstrual Cycles

Birth control pills are commonly prescribed to help a woman normalize her menstrual cycle. The pills, which contain the hormones estrogen and progestin in varying amounts, work to even out your estrogen and progesterone levels while also lowering androgen levels. If a woman responds well to the drugs, the result is a regular period with lighter bleeding. And because the birth control pills bring hormones into balance, they also can help prevent acne and excess growth of body hair.

Oral contraceptives come in three basic types: *monophasic*, *biphasic*, and *triphasic*. The pills are color-coded to prevent confusion. A monophasic pill provides a level daily dose of the hormones estrogen and progestin. For twenty-one days, you take the same strength of both hormones (one color); then for seven days, you take inactive tablets (another color); to complete your twenty-eight-day cycle. The inactive tablets are included so that women do not get out of the habit of taking a pill daily.

With biphasics, the estrogen level stays the same, but the progestin level is increased in the later part of the cycle. The reason for this variation is to try to more closely mimic a woman's natural cycle. If you are using a biphasic twenty-one-day pill, you will take tablets of one strength (color) during the first part of your cycle and tablets of a second strength (color) during the second part of your cycle. The exact number of days you will take each strength varies depending on the medication, but it will always add up to twenty-one days. With a twenty-eight-day biphasic prescription, during the last seven days of your cycle you will take a third colored pill that is hormonally inactive.

Triphasic pills are designed to most closely mimic the natural menstrual cycle. If you are using a triphasic twenty-one-day pill, you will take three varying doses of hormones, with each pill a different color. The number of days at each dosing level varies from five to ten, depending on the prescription. With a twenty-eight-day triphasic prescription, you will take an additional seven inactive tablets, which are a fourth color.

Some women respond well to birth control pills. As Missy, age twenty-two, explained, "I am taking a combination pill, with both estrogen and progesterone (progestin). I took one for years that was just the progesterone type and it worked well, but after the birth of my twins, it wasn't strong enough. I seemed to bleed and spot all month. I switched three months ago, and so far so good. I have stopped losing hair on my head, and I have stopped growing hair where I don't want it. My cycles are also right on time. I have always had good luck with birth control pills for controlling PCOS symptoms."

Birth Control Pills

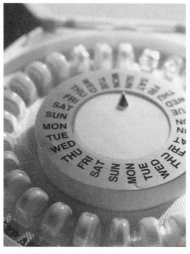

Oral contraceptives help to normalize hormone levels, often resulting in regular menstrual cycles and the lessening of other PCOS symptoms such as acne and excess body hair.

Yet some women have reported a worsening of PCOS symptoms while taking triphasics. The first phase has such a low estrogen dose that it may not properly suppress the growth of cysts and other PCOS symptoms, and it may well exacerbate the symptoms. There may be other reasons that haven't yet been fully explored.

"The first pill I was on was triphasic," said Shelly, age twenty-nine. "It was great for four years, and then I started having mood swings. I had a lot of stress in my life at that time, which the doctor said could have contributed to the new PMS (premenstrual syndrome) symptoms. He switched me to a monophasic pill. The mood swings went away, but my periods were extremely heavy, requiring changes of a maximum tampon with pad backup every two hours. When I became anemic about a year later, I switched types of pills again and tolerated them well."

Choosing an Oral Contraceptive

Experiences with oral contraceptives can vary widely from woman to woman. The effects of birth control pills on our bodies are complex, and there are many individual variations in the effects on PCOS. Accordingly, there is no uniform birth control regimen to manage PCOS symptoms. The best advice is to proceed with caution.

If you are on an oral contraceptive, make sure your doctor is monitoring you closely. If you think the pills are worsening your condition, such as causing breakthrough bleeding or making your acne worse, tell your doctor right away. Your physician may switch you to another type of pill. If you were prescribed an oral contraceptive in the past and did not do well with it, let your physician know.

Side Effects of Oral Contraceptives

Generally, birth control medications are safe and, for most women, taking oral contraceptives does not create problems. The dosages in birth control pills today are significantly lower than when they were first introduced in the 1960s. As a result, women have fewer side effects. If side effects do occur, it is usually during the first three months of use. Check with your doctor as soon as possible if any of the following side effects occur:

- Changes in the uterine bleeding pattern at menses or between menses
- Decreased bleeding at menses
- Breakthrough bleeding or spotting between periods
- Prolonged bleeding at menses
- An occasional stopping of menstrual bleeding
- A complete stopping of menstrual bleeding that occurs several months in a row

Less-common side effects include headaches or migraines, increased blood pressure, and vaginal infection with vaginal itching or irritation.

Other side effects may occur but usually diminish as your body adjusts to the medication. However, check with your doctor if any of the following side effects persist:

- Abdominal cramping or bloating
- Acne (usually less common after the first three months and may improve if it already exists)
- Breast pain, tenderness, or swelling
- Dizziness
- Nausea
- Vomiting

- Brown, blotchy spots on exposed skin
- Gain or loss of body or facial hair
- Increased or decreased interest in sexual intercourse
- Increased sensitivity of skin to sunlight
- Weight gain or loss

For some women with special health problems, oral contraceptives can cause more-serious side effects. These can include noncancerous liver tumors, blood clots, or related problems, such as a stroke. The following side effects may be caused by blood clots. Get emergency help immediately if any of the following side effects occur:

- Abdominal or stomach pain (sudden, severe, or continuing)
- Coughing up blood
- Headache (severe or sudden)
- Loss of coordination (sudden)
- Change in or loss of vision (sudden)
- Pains in chest, groin, or leg (especially in calf of leg)
- Shortness of breath (sudden or unexplained)
- Slurring of speech (sudden)
- Weakness, numbness, or pain in arm or leg (unexplained)

Although these side effects are rare, they can be serious enough to cause death. Risks also increase with age and from smoking cigarettes. If you are a smoker, you should not take birth control pills after the age of thirty-five.

Drugs to Induce Menstruation

Many women with PCOS take medications monthly to induce their periods. However, these medications do not cause ovulation. If you wish to become pregnant, it will likely be necessary to take other medications that promote ovulation. Still, it is possible to become pregnant while using period-inducing medications if you ovulate spontaneously. The two most common medications that induce menstruation are *medroxyprogesterone acetate (MPA)* and progesterone.

MPA (Provera)

The drug MPA is a synthetic medication that mimics the action of the natural hormone progesterone to induce a period. The commonly prescribed form of this drug is *Provera.* If your estrogen levels are adequate, your period should begin within one week after completing the medication. If your period does not begin, talk to your physician. Some women begin menstruating while they are in the middle of taking this medication. If this occurs, speak to your doctor about stopping the medication.

Normal Ovary

Polycystic Ovary

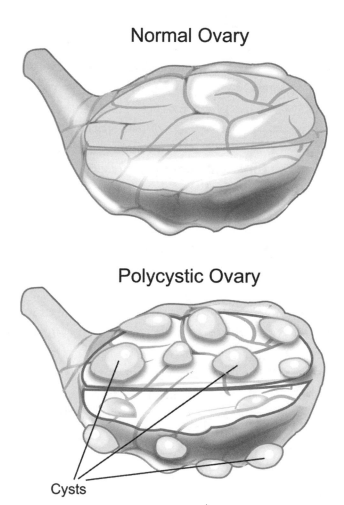

Cysts

The normal ovary, above, has a smooth contour. The ovary below shows cysts, which result from the follicle not releasing an egg each month. As this process repeats, multiple follicles build up, forming a cyst.

Progesterone (Prometrium)

Taken orally, progesterone, sold as *Prometrium*, also can help start the menstrual cycle. It is not a synthetic drug; rather, it is a natural progesterone that originates from a plant extract. It is similar to the body's natural progesterone. Prometrium is reported to have fewer side effects than Provera, although some women cannot tolerate either. Side effects may include abdominal cramping, back pain, bloating, and breast tenderness.

PCOS Symptom: Enlarged Ovaries

Approximately 70 percent of women with PCOS have cysts on their ovaries. Cysts occur naturally on the ovaries each month when follicles containing an egg develop and rupture, releasing an egg. These cysts can reach a diameter of two to four inches but usually disappear with menstruation. However, women with PCOS have multiple follicles that never mature and never rupture to release the egg in a regular fashion. As this process repeats month after month, multiple follicles form. The ovaries can become enlarged, taking on a thick, shiny, white coating, sometimes referred to as an "oyster shell." In women with many cysts, the cysts are said to resemble "strands of pearls" draped over their ovaries.

Treatment for Enlarged Ovaries

If you have ovarian cysts and you're trying to get pregnant, the goal of treatment is to cause the cysts to mature and release an egg so you can conceive. The fertility drug Clomid is commonly the first line of treatment for women with PCOS who want to get pregnant. More information on getting pregnant is available in chapter 5.

If you're not trying to get pregnant, PCOS treatment is not focused on the ovarian cysts. Instead, the treatment is focused on minimizing the PCOS symptoms with drugs, such as insulin sensitizers and oral contraceptives.

PCOS Symptom: Weight Gain

Not all women with PCOS struggle with their weight. In fact being overweight is not a true symptom of PCOS; however, being overweight and obesity is associated with PCOS. Nearly half the women with PCOS are obese.

Insulin resistance, common with PCOS, also causes the production of more male hormones, which also contributes to weight gain. Another troublesome thing about insulin resistance is that once you eat carbohydrates and the insulin has finished its job of storing them, the body doesn't sit dormant waiting for more. Instead, it rushes a signal to the brain, giving out false hunger pains. Naturally, you eat more to satisfy your hunger, and the vicious cycle continues. With each dose of carbohydrates, you produce more and more insulin, causing hunger signals each time. This explains why you can become hungry one to three

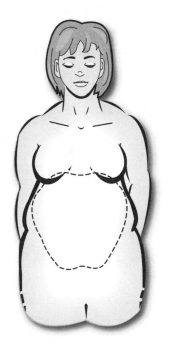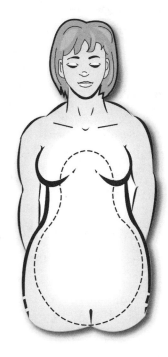

Women with PCOS who gain weight tend to accumulate the extra weight in the waist, giving them the "apple shape." The waist is larger than the hips.

When women who do not have PCOS gain weight, they typically accumulate the excess weight in the hips, giving them more of a "pear shape."

hours after eating a satisfying meal and why a sugary dessert can make you feel hungry again.

Weight gain in women with PCOS tends to result in an "apple-shaped" body, with the waist being thicker than the hips. This is more typical of a male-pattern weight gain. Weight gain in a woman without PCOS tends to result in a "pear-shaped" body, with the extra weight at the hips, buttocks, and thighs, while the waist remains thinner. Research shows that women with apple-shaped bodies tend to experience more health problems, including cardiovascular disease and diabetes.

Losing Weight

Losing weight is one of the best treatments for overweight women with PCOS. It helps to lower the level of insulin in the body and indirectly reduces the body's production of testosterone, alleviating many of the PCOS symptoms. Losing weight reduces the risk of cardiovascular disease and Type 2 diabetes. It also boosts one's energy level and self-confidence. "When you have PCOS," explained Cori, age thirty-four, "you think more about how you feel about your body. Your relationship with your body is horrible."

Low-Carb Diets

Because the connection between PCOS and insulin resistance is so strong, many women have successfully lost weight by watching their carbohydrate intake, especially when other types of diets have failed. When fewer carbohydrates are coming in, your insulin and glucose levels drop and your body can actually burn fat for energy. This is what causes you to lose weight. "For the first time in my life, I was successful at dieting with a low-carbohydrate food plan," said Diana, age twenty-nine. "I lost weight and I lost the cravings I had when my blood sugar dropped. When I go off 'low-carbing,' then my weight creeps back on, so I know this has to be a long-term commitment."

Increasingly, a low-carbohydrate diet is being touted as one of the best ways for women to lose weight. There are many popular low-carbohydrate diets. Some are more restrictive than others, so you might have to try several until you find one that you can stick to and that is effective for you. For instance, you may decide to follow one of the popular low-carbohydrate, high-protein diets. Such diets recommend cutting your intake of carbohydrates to thirty grams or less a day.

Once you have reached your goal weight, then you gradually increase your carbohydrates until you stop losing weight. Some women swear by it, but others find this type of diet too restrictive and difficult to maintain. There is some controversy over whether low-carb diets, which permit high fat intake, are healthful.

On the other hand, if you cannot totally give up carbohydrates, one of the less-restrictive plans might be for you. Typically, no snacks are allowed, and two of your meals must be extremely low in carbohydrates. However, you are allowed one meal in which you can eat a moderate portion of carbohydrates. These diets are based on the theory that your body is primed on how much insulin to release based upon previous meals. So, with two meals of low carbohydrates and one meal of moderate carbohydrates, your body is tricked into releasing more insulin. Therefore, you store less fat and have steadier blood sugar levels.

Some women have successfully designed their own "moderated-carbohydrate" eating plans. You can create your own style of restricting your carbohydrate intake by eating mostly meats, eggs, cheeses, and vegetables. Foods high in carbohydrates are restricted as much as possible. Foods that tend to be high in carbohydrates include, but are not limited to, breads, cakes, cereal, chips, chocolate, cookies, crackers, fruit, ice cream, juice, pasta, potatoes, pretzels, rice, pie, popcorn, and sodas.

Exercise

Exercise is an essential treatment for women with PCOS. It can help women in several ways. Exercise plays an important part in weight loss. It has been proven to help achieve proper insulin levels, which, in turn, affect hormone levels. In addition, exercise helps you feel good about your body and gives you a sense of accomplishment.

Cori, age thirty-two, who jogs every other day and weight-trains on alternate days, knows that not all women with PCOS are able or willing to jog three miles at a stretch. "We all just need to move, whether it is yoga or water aerobics or walking. Exercising has changed my life."

PCOS Symptom: Acne

Adult acne is another particularly annoying problem for women with PCOS. It develops on the face, chest, and back. Acne forms when male hormones increase *sebum,* a combination of skin oils and old skin tissue, which clogs pores. Then, bacteria that thrive on sebum grow, resulting in pimples—whiteheads and blackheads.

Treatment for Acne

As noted earlier, the hormone balance brought on by birth control pills can help reduce the occurrence of acne. There are also other treatment options. If you decide to see a dermatologist about your acne, he/she might prescribe topical treatments. One such treatment is a drug called *adapalene (Differin).* It works by keeping the pores open. It's available as a cream, gel, or solution. Another topical treatment, *tretinoin,* a cream sold as *Retin-A,* works by promoting skin cell turnover, eliminating the oil and debris that may clog pores.

Some women's acne improves with oral antibiotics such as *tetracycline* or *erythromycin,* or a combination of both. For more-severe acne, the dermatologist might prescribe *Accutane (isotretinoin),* a potent oral medicine that reduces the amount of oil produced by the oil glands, allowing the skin to clear up. The drug *spironolactone (Aldactone),* prescribed for excess body hair, can also help eliminate acne since it reduces the buildup of oil in the pores.

Note that Accutane and spironolactone should not be used if you are pregnant or planning to become pregnant; these drugs may cause birth defects. Retin-A cream should also be avoided since the absorbed cream can enter the mother's bloodstream and be passed into breast milk.

Cleansing the Skin

In addition to topical preparations and oral medications, women with PCOS are encouraged to take good care of their skin. The following skin care guidelines can help:

- Clean the skin gently but thoroughly with soap and water, removing all dirt or makeup. Wash as often as needed, at least daily and after exercising, to control oil. Use a clean washcloth every day to prevent bacterial reinfection.

- Use steam or a warm, moist compress to open clogged pores.

- Shampoo hair daily when possible. Use a dandruff shampoo if necessary.

- Comb or pull hair back to keep it out of the face.

- Use topical astringents to remove excess oil.

- Don't squeeze, scratch, pick, or rub lesions. These activities can increase skin damage. Wash your hands before and after caring for skin lesions to reduce the chance of infection.

- Use oil-free skin care products or those that do not clog pores.

- Don't rest your face on your hands. This irritates the skin of the face.

Acne can also be treated with over-the-counter medications that help cleanse the skin.

PCOS Symptom: Acanthosis Nigricans

Another skin problem that affects some women with PCOS is *acanthosis nigricans*, a disorder that causes light-brown-to-black, velvety patches of skin on the back and sides of the neck. It can also occur under the arms and in the groin. This skin disorder is sometimes referred to as "dirty skin" since women say that their skin looks "dirty." Acanthosis nigricans may begin at any age and may appear gradually over a period of years.

Treatment for Acanthosis Nigricans

It appears there is an association between insulin resistance and acanthosis nigricans; often, the dark patches of skin will fade when underlying problems, such as insulin resistance and obesity, are treated. It may take months or years, however, for this to resolve.

Prescriptions that may provide some improvement for this condition include topical solutions such as Retin-A, alpha hydroxy acid, and salicylic acid; these mild acids have long been used to rejuvenate facial skin. Some women respond to the oral medication Accutane. You may also want to talk to a dermatologist about dermabrasion or laser therapy that may help reduce the thickness of skin in the affected areas.

When acanthosis nigricans develops, a medical evaluation should also be done to determine whether an endocrine gland disorder, such as an insulin-secreting tumor, has developed.

PCOS Symptom: Skin Tags

In addition to adult acne, women with PCOS often experience other skin problems, including skin tags. Also called *acrochordons*, skin tags are teardrop-shaped pieces of skin that are usually found in the armpits and around the neck but can also occur on the chest and back, and under the breasts, or in the groin area. Skin tags are often about the size of a pin-

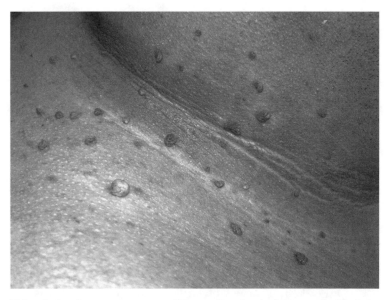

This photo shows a woman with acanthosis nigricans and skin tags around her neck. Both of these conditions are associated with insulin resistance. *Photo courtesy of Dermnetnz.org.*

head but can be as large as a raisin. They are benign growths and are usually painless, except for occasional irritation from rubbing by clothing or other friction. Their origin is unknown. They are thought to be a symptom of insulin resistance.

"I have skin tags appear two or three at a time," explained Michelle, age thirty-eight. "One time I tied dental floss around one and tightened it every day until it fell off, but then it got infected and I had to go to the doctor. I heard of another woman who just cut it off, but her armpit was swollen for a week. Now, my dermatologist removes them. This is the safe way to handle skin tags."

Treatment for Skin Tags

The safest and most effective treatment for skin tags is removal by a physician. He or she may cut them off with a scalpel or scissors or remove them with either freezing or electrosurgery—burning them off with electric current.

Generally, this procedure would be considered cosmetic, and insurance would not pay for it. However, insurance will usually pay for the procedure if you explain to the physician that the condition is irritated by your bra strap or from wearing jewelry.

PCOS Symptom: Excess Body Hair

One of the more-difficult cosmetic symptoms of PCOS is hirsutism, excess hair growth on the body. The increase in body hair is caused by excess levels of

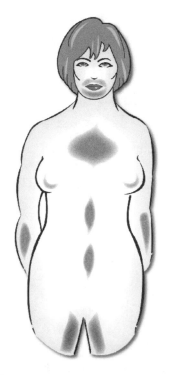

Excess body hair is one of the cosmetic symptoms of PCOS. Dark hair often appears in the shaded areas shown above—upper lip, chin, chest, arms, breasts, stomach, and thighs.

the male hormone androgen in the body. This unwanted hair usually grows above the lip or on the chin. It also grows thicker than usual on the limbs. There may also be hair on the chest or an extension of pubic hair on the abdomen and thighs. Such increased hair growth is usually noted in the late teen years and gradually increases as a woman gets older.

"The hirsutism is embarrassing because it is such an outward, masculine sign," explained Beth, age thirty-five. "For me, it became a problem at age twelve. I started shaving after a particularly cruel comment from a junior high school boy. I have shaved ever since. I also remove hair on my chest, breasts, and stomach in addition to my armpits and legs. It even grows on the top side of my fingers."

There are a variety of hair removal methods. You may wish to use one or a combination, depending on your needs and skin sensitivity.

Treatment for Excess Body Hair

Oral Contraceptives

As mentioned, oral contraceptives can help stabilize a woman's hormone levels, often reducing her level of male hormones, such as testosterone. The reduction in male hormones inhibits the excessive hair growth. Oral contraceptives won't make existing hair go away, but they will slow the growth of new hair.

Laser Therapy

Laser hair removal is offered by many medical offices, salons, and day spas. The FDA does not permit laser manufacturers to claim that laser treatment is permanent or painless, but they are permitted to advertise long-term results for hair removal. Laser treatment is a relatively fast route to temporarily removing hair, but it is rarely permanent. Lasered hair often returns in three to six months. The treatment is most effective in people with light skin and dark hair; it is usually ineffective on gray, red, or blond hair. Laser treatment carries a risk of scarring around the treated area.

Lasers must be used only by a licensed practitioner. Both the practitioner and the patient should wear protective goggles. The key to the effectiveness of the laser is proper adjustment of the pulse-width—the amount of time the laser is on and able to pass through the skin to reach the hair follicle. At the follicle level, the laser energy is absorbed and transformed into heat that disables the follicle. As a result, hair growth is impaired without affecting surrounding tissue. Each laser pulse treats about a one-half-inch area, which can contain ten or more hairs. The amount of time the treatment takes depends on the size of the area to be treated. Some lasers can treat an entire leg in half an hour and the upper lip in sixty seconds.

Since some follicles can go dormant and produce hair at different times, several visits may be necessary for total treatment. Your physician will work with you to develop the optimal treatment strategy.

Most patients describe the treatment as feeling like a series of rubber band snaps to the skin. The majority of patients tolerate this sensation without anesthetics. However, for patient comfort, topical anesthetics or oral sedatives may be used. Within about thirty minutes of treatment, the skin may become pink or red, and it may feel like a mild sunburn for a day or so. Newer lasers are more efficient and cause less skin discoloration.

Electrolysis

With professional *electrolysis,* a technician called an electrologist inserts a small probe along each hair, and a small electrical discharge destroys the hair follicle. This method may result in permanent hair loss, but it takes time. Only a small area is treated every few weeks. To complete treatment in one area can take months.

There are risks with electrolysis. Scarring of the skin and electric shock can occur if the technician is unskilled. Other risks include infection that can be caused by an unsterilized needle. Many states require licensing, and you should seek a qualified individual to perform this procedure.

Let your electrologist know if you have any medical problems. Mention your PCOS and any medications you are taking. "My electrologist asks what medication I am on and writes a report on the hair growth for my doctor. She documents such things as new hair growth, how the treatments are keeping up with my hair growth, my mood, how my complexion looks, and whether she notices any weight gain or loss," explained Wanda, age thirty-four. A good electrologist will also give you a short lesson on how hair grows.

According to Sara, age thirty-five, "I've been going for electrolysis for twelve years. I started with my chin and neck. It took a long time to get it under control. Now the hair on my chin is gone, except for two, which take about six to seven weeks to grow back. The remaining hair on my neck is very light and blends in with my skin, except for several dark hairs that grow back every five to six weeks. The hair on my stomach bothers me, but not as much as the hair on my arms. So two years ago, I started electrolysis on both forearms. The hair has thinned, but is still dark.

Electrolysis isn't for everyone, and it does involve needles. It takes time and patience and can be expensive. But for me it is worth it."

If you go to an electrologist, ask if he/she is a certified professional electrologist (CPE). Certification means the electrologist has gone through a voluntary testing program with the American Electrology Association, which also requires continuing education. Also ask about his/her training and experience and whether disposable, sterile needles are used. Make sure the technician wears gloves.

Anti-Androgen Medication

The medication spironolactone, (Aldactone) is actually a diuretic that is prescribed for those with hypertension. However, it also fights the effects of androgens in the skin and can slowly reduce excessive hair growth. This medication is often combined with an oral contraceptive. The contraceptive usually contains both estrogen and progesterone, hormones that may also help reduce excessive hair by stabilizing female hormone levels. Talk with your doctor about trying combinations of these drugs.

"I've been on Aldactone for over two years and find it works really well for me," said Diana, age twenty-two. "I used to wax the hair above my upper lip, and now I pull only a few stray hairs with the tweezers once a month. The excess hair on other areas has also slowed to nearly nothing. The Aldactone also cleared up my complexion and knocked out the serious water retention problems I was having. If you use this drug, you have to stick with it. It takes a few months to really kick in, and all the symptoms come rushing back when you stop taking it."

The adverse effects of the usage of this drug include upset stomach, thirst, excessive urination, nausea, headaches, weakness, breast tenderness, reduced libido, sensitivity to sunlight, and excess levels of potassium in the blood. Some women report that spironolactone has thrown their menstrual cycles off and has caused lightheadedness. This drug may also be associated with birth defects and should be avoided by women attempting pregnancy or who are pregnant.

The drug *flutamide (Eulexin)* decreases a cell's ability to bind androgens. Consequently, it may decrease the symptoms of PCOS, specifically excess hair growth. It has not been approved by the FDA for this use, however. Due to the risk of toxicity to the liver, this drug is rarely prescribed for women with PCOS.

Depilatory Creams

Over-the-counter depilatory creams act like a chemical razor blade. They are also available as lotions, gels, aerosols, and roll-ons. A thick layer is applied to the skin for fifteen to thirty minutes, then wiped off, taking the hair with it. However, the creams can irritate the skin. It is important to read directions carefully because some creams are formulated only for certain areas of the body. Also, they should never be used on the eyebrows, or on broken or inflamed skin.

Prescription Cream

Approved by the FDA, *Vaniqa* is the first prescription cream reported to reduce excessive facial hair in women. The cream is applied to the face, like a moisturizer, twice a day. It works by blocking the enzyme that makes the hair follicles grow. It takes about eight weeks for the cream to work. Vaniqa must be used regularly, or hair growth will resume. During the clinical trials for the cream, most women had no major side effects; some women reported slight skin irritation such as redness, stinging, or rash on the site where the cream was applied. Only 2 percent of the women discontinued the trial.

Shaving

Shaving is by far the most common method of hair removal. Shaving twice a day, if necessary, will prevent unsightly stubble. A clean razor with a sharp blade is essential for a safe and comfortable shave. Skin should never be shaved dry; wet hair is pliable and easier to cut. Contrary to popular opinion, shaving does not make the hair grow in thicker or change the rate of hair growth.

Tweezing and Waxing

Tweezing and waxing may be more painful than using a depilatory, but the results are longer lasting, and without strong chemical odors. However, tweezing is impractical for large areas because it is a slow and painful process. It is mostly done for facial hair.

Waxing involves applying melted wax to the skin. After the wax hardens, it is stripped off, and hairs are pulled out by the roots. A small area should be tested before doing a large area.

Waxing needs to be repeated every six weeks on the face, legs, underarms, and bikini areas. Waxes may be hot or cold, and may contain combinations of such ingredients as paraffin and beeswax, oils or fats, and a resin that makes the wax adhere to the skin. Waxing can be done in a beauty salon or at home. Some women have their own recipes for "sugaring," a home-made wax made with sugar and lemon juice. Some suggest waxing should only be done by an expert to limit the chance of infection.

If you're taking the drug Accutane, avoid waxing until you've been off the drug for thirty days. This drug can make your skin fragile and susceptible to tearing when the wax is peeled off.

Bleaching

Bleaching doesn't remove the hair, but makes it lighter and less obvious. Some women, however, do not like the way it looks when it grows back half blond, half dark. For women with dark hair, it may look unusual to have blond body hair. Women with sensitive skin may have a reaction to the bleaching chemicals, and some women may dislike the odor of the chemicals in the removers.

PCOS Symptom: Thinning Hair

In some women, hair loss, or *androgenic alopecia*, results in loss of hair all over the head. It is an unwelcome reminder of living with PCOS. The hair loss is likely due to an increase in androgens, the male hormones. With alopecia, hairs become smaller and smaller during each growth phase. Hair usually thins the most on the top of the head, the part of the scalp that is most androgen sensitive. Frontal balding and hairline recession is seen only in the most severe cases.

Treatment for Thinning Hair

The topical medication *minoxidil* is the most widely recommended treatment for male-pattern baldness. Sold as *Rogaine*, the drug appears to work by gradually enlarging and lengthening hair follicles that have been gradually shrinking. The growth phase may also be extended, giving the hairs an opportunity to lengthen before they fall out. It takes about three to four months of use to see evidence of any regrowth and up to six months to determine whether minoxidil will be beneficial.

Minoxidil must be used continually. Once discontinued, any new hair growth will not continue. Minoxidil may exceed the budgets of some individuals; however, a generic version is less expensive. Because these drugs are considered cosmetic treatments, their cost is usually not covered by health insurance.

Another drug, Retin-A, also used as a topical treatment for acne and other skin disorders, can be used alone or in combination with minoxidil. Retin-A has been known to produce moderate to good hair growth in individuals with male-pattern baldness and *alopecia areata*, a condition that causes patches of baldness. If a combination is used, it is suggested that minoxidil be applied in the morning and a Retin-A gel in the evening to reduce the problem of skin sensitivity to sunlight.

PCOS Symptom: Depression

Although depression is not an actual symptom of PCOS, it is often associated with PCOS. It's possible that the hormonal problems brought on by PCOS cause depression; it's also possible that PCOS symptoms such as weight gain and infertility cause depression. Most researchers do agree that a woman's physiology, which is so closely related to hormone fluctuations, is an important key to understanding depression. Hormones influence our behavior as well as our health in complex ways still not completely understood by medical science.

Depression associated with PCOS is discussed more fully in chapter 4.

Hysterectomy Is Not a Solution

Finally, it's important to note that a *hysterectomy*, or surgical removal of the uterus, is not an appropriate medical treatment for PCOS. Unfortunately, physicians who are not knowledgeable about current PCOS treatment options may recommend a hysterectomy. If your physician suggests hysterectomy for PCOS, it is important to seek a second opinion. You'll want to gain a full understanding of exactly why this surgery is being suggested and why other treatment options are not being recommended.

4

Coping Emotionally with PCOS

"**I** often ask, Why me? Why do any of us have PCOS?" said Nan, a thirty-six-year-old woman with PCOS.

"I have a hard time accepting the fact that I simply had some 'genetic bad luck,' and that I cannot fix it. I worry that it may be taking a toll on my heart, and it has certainly taken an emotional toll. How do I hang on? How do I manage?"

Depression

PCOS can be frightening, overwhelming, and discouraging. Fear about health issues, grief about a loss of control over family planning, and anger at years of misdiagnosis are all common reactions. Women can suffer depression as a side effect of PCOS, or they may feel depressed because of PCOS-related difficulties. Depression can manifest itself in physical symptoms such as:

- Headaches
- Stomach problems

- Insomnia
- Loss of, or sudden increase in appetite
- Sudden change in menstruation

Emotional symptoms may include feelings of:

- Emptiness
- Sadness
- Hopelessness
- Guilt
- Remorse

Cognitive or behavioral changes may also occur, including:

- Loss of concentration
- Memory loss
- Lack of libido
- Inability to respond sexually

Some women with PCOS remember being depressed even in childhood.

"I can look at myself in pictures from an early age and see an enormous sadness, even at age four," said Nina, a thirty-five-year-old with PCOS. "By my early twenties, I felt as though I was going insane. My body was so out of whack, and it was crying out for help. I always felt as though there was a black cloud over me."

Depression and Infertility

Infertility is a difficult emotional hurdle. PCOS robs a woman of many things—perhaps cruelest of all, her ability to conceive naturally and build a family. Many women first learn that they have PCOS because they have sought the help of a fertility specialist. By that time, they typically have been trying to get pregnant for a year or more. Infertility alone is a particularly trying experience, but combined with PCOS, it can be traumatic. And discovering that you are at elevated risk for life-threatening medical conditions is also frightening. The good news is, the more we learn about PCOS, the more tools we have to restore fertility and to avoid potential complications such as heart disease, cancer, and diabetes.

Treatment for Depression

Depression can be treated a number of ways. Often, the expression of thoughts and emotions through talk therapy with a professional therapist can help. Some individuals may benefit from counseling in a group setting, where they feel less isolated and benefit from the experiences of others.

Prescription antidepressants are also frequently used to treat clinical depression and may be an appropriate choice. There are no specific antidepressants used for patients with PCOS. Women may have to try a variety of antidepressants before they find the one that works best for them.

"I have had to accept the fact that my hormonal changes wreak havoc with my moods and well-being if I don't intervene with an antidepressant," said Susan, age thirty-six.

"I am simply not willing to feel depressed. I take a low-dose antidepressant and am grateful to have my 'real' personality back. I'm more positive, creative, and focused, and a lot less worried."

Nevertheless, women are sometimes afraid of being diagnosed as depressed. They may not want it in their medical records, or they are concerned that needing an antidepressant is somehow a weakness.

"The stigmas about depression/anxiety and medication are finally shifting away in our society. I look forward to the day when, like diabetics and heart disease patients, people with depression can be treated openly without shame. Depression can require medications, just like other illnesses," said Nancy.

Embarrassment

Side effects such as acne, hirsutism, and obesity can cause women to feel less than feminine and bring up issues about self-worth. Our culture unrealistically expects all women should be thin and have flawless skin and smooth, hairless bodies. Women with PCOS may not look like that ideal and may feel ashamed of the way they look. Some women are reluctant for partners to see them nude because of their weight. Embarrassment from physical symptoms as well as the difficulty of living with infertility can leave women feeling isolated and withdrawn.

Stress and Anxiety

Stress is defined as a feeling of tension that is both emotional and physical. Women with PCOS may experience stress about infertility treatment, health-care choices or expenses, or the reality of living with a chronic illness. Stress management is intended to help reduce tension. It involves making emotional and physical changes. The degree of stress and the desire to make the changes will determine the level of change required.

One's attitude plays an important role. It can influence whether a situation is stressful. A person with a negative attitude will often perceive many situations as stressful. Negative attitude is a predictor of stress.

Physical well-being is an important part of controlling our moods. If our nutrition is poor, our bodies are stressed and we are not able to respond well to stressful situations. As a result, we can be more susceptible to infections. Poor nutrition can be related to unhealthy food choices, inadequate food intake, or an erratic eating schedule. A nutritionally unbalanced eating pattern also means an inadequate intake of nutrients. Inadequate physical activity can further result in a stressful state for the body. A consistent program of physical activity can contribute to a sense of well-being.

"I can't say this enough—even simple walking is a good stress releaser. Add it to your routine. Not only will it help increase your utilization of excess insulin and androgens, it will also help you deal with stress and will help relieve depression, too!" said Rebecca, age thirty-two.

Tips for Stress Relief

You can begin to relieve stress by working on developing a positive attitude. Refocus negative thoughts into positive ones. Talk positively to yourself. The following guidelines can also help you reduce stress.

Physical activity:
- Start an individualized program of physical activity.
- Decide on a specific time, type, frequency, and level of physical activity.

Nutrition:
- Eat foods that will improve your health and well-being.
- Eat an appropriate amount of food on a reasonable schedule.

Social support:
- Make an effort to interact socially with people.
- Reach out to individuals.
- Nurture yourself and others.
- Plan some fun events.

Relaxation:
- Use relaxation techniques (guided imagery, listening to music, prayer, etc.). Learn about and try different techniques, then choose one or two that work for you.
- Take time for personal interests and hobbies.
- Listen to your body.
- Take a mini-retreat.

If you're unable to manage stress, consider the help of a licensed social worker or psychotherapist who can help. Scheduling time with one of these professionals is often helpful in learning stress management strategies and relaxation techniques.

Finding Support

We need people in our lives who cherish us, support us, and encourage us. If we do not have such people, we need to actively seek them out. They might be in your family, church, or place of employment. If you are trying to conceive, your reproductive specialist will often have a professional counselor who can meet with you; you might also consider contacting a support organization such as RESOLVE, the national infertility association and a valuable information source for more than 7 million women and men coping with infertility.

Professional Support

Professional support is provided by both medical practitioners and mental health experts. The first line of defense is a good doctor who not only diagnoses your problem but also treats you with understanding and works with you to find solutions to your problems. However, for many women, this alone is not enough; they benefit from sharing their feelings and experiences with other women who are dealing with the same problems.

Peer Support

The emotional support from others who have PCOS is invaluable. Peer support offers the ability to talk freely about the issues you have been dealing with. It can be especially wonderful to talk with others who have firsthand knowledge of what you are going through. Sharing with others can lighten the load.

One source of peer support is the Polycystic Ovarian Syndrome Association (PCOSA), an international support and education organization for women with PCOS. The organization has several different avenues for peer support, including local chapters and Internet forums. Many women who participate in the chapters and forums find this to be one of the best forms of therapy. Person-to-person support is provided through the network of local chapters.

PCOSA offers information for women who want children, those who are not trying to conceive, teens, women in menopause, and general PCOS support. To subscribe to an online e-mail support group, you can log on to the PCOSA Web page and enroll at www.pcosupport.org. You can choose to have each e-mail delivered as it arrives, or in digest form, as one complete package daily. Bulletin boards do not involve e-mail but allow you to post or respond to topics regarding PCOS. Like the mailing lists, they offer discussions on a number of different topics.

Family and Friends

It is usually a relief to finally know that the odd constellation of symptoms you experience is attributable to one medically recognized disorder. The next problem is, do you share that information with your partner, family, and/or friends? If so, how? It is especially important that you help those who live with you understand PCOS and what it is doing to your body. Once they understand how PCOS affects you, they can be active participants in your healing. Your partner may be able to shed insight or help you identify patterns.

Family and friends can offer support by learning more about PCOS, attending PCOS support group meetings, encouraging healthy choices, and simply asking what they can do to help.

5

Getting Pregnant

For years, Mary had dreamed of becoming a mom. Even as a little girl, she loved to rock her baby brother and sing him to sleep. She was the most sought-after babysitter on the block as she grew older. But now, at age forty-one, being around babies makes her sad. It's a painful reminder that she and her husband are still childless.

Mary had three years of fertility treatment managed by her gynecologist, who tried repeated rounds of medication without success. It wasn't until she decided to go to a reproductive endocrinologist that she was diagnosed with PCOS. Together, they agreed she had other treatment options. Mary is still waiting but is feeling more hopeful now that she has found a fertility specialist.

Mary is not alone. Infertility strikes about one in seven couples trying to become pregnant.

Infertility and PCOS

PCOS is one of the leading causes of infertility. Many women with PCOS have difficulty becoming pregnant due to their irregular menstrual cycles, or lack of cycles. Irregular cycles can make it extremely difficult to pinpoint when or if ovulation is occurring. Fortunately, some women with PCOS who do occasionally ovulate can become pregnant without fertility treatments. Overall, even though some women with PCOS are unable to become pregnant, a great number of women do conceive and have successful pregnancies, either on their own or by undergoing fertility treatments.

Life Style Changes

Life style changes, such as losing weight and exercising, may increase the chances for pregnancy in women with PCOS. Weight loss can make periods more regular. There may be a role for bariatric (weight loss) surgery and the use of drugs that induce weight loss for the treatment of obesity in PCOS; however, these approaches are newer and large clinical trials are needed in these areas. It is important to receive counseling prior to conception in order to identify risk factors for reproductive failure and to correct them prior to any fertility treatment.

Choosing a Fertility Specialist

Within the last decade, many strides have been made to help women conceive. In fact, two-thirds of those seeking medical help are eventually able to conceive. If you decide to seek medical help, one of the first steps to successfully managing your fertility treatments is finding a good physician. You want to find a fertility specialist—someone who primarily treats women and couples with fertility problems. Most likely, this will be a reproductive endocrinologist (RE).

An RE is usually trained as an OB/GYN and has received additional training in reproductive endocrinology. When choosing an RE, look for one who is board certified and who has completed a two- to three-year fellowship in reproductive endocrinology, a specialty in which the physician focuses specifically on how hormones affect reproduction and pregnancy. He/she should be very knowledgeable about PCOS and be thorough, attentive, and compassionate with you and your mate.

A fertility specialist should want to talk with you extensively before beginning any treatment, to find out both your and your partner's medical history and your overall goals for achieving pregnancy. He/she should also be available to answer any questions and concerns as they come up. Furthermore, since fertility, especially ovulation, can be somewhat unpredictable, you may want to find someone with weekend and/or evening office hours so that if you experience complications or need to go in for testing, you can be seen right away.

Below are a few other questions you should consider before selecting a fertility specialist:

- **Who is recommending the specialist?** Make sure whoever is recommending the fertility specialist is reputable and qualified to make such a recommendation. If you have a good OB/GYN or family physician, he/she is most likely qualified to help you find an appropriate fertility specialist.

- **What is the specialist's background?** Ask if the fertility specialist is board certified and how many years he/she has been working with patients having difficulty conceiving, especially those with PCOS. Also, you might want to ask your fertility specialist about his/her pregnancy rates as well as live birth and multiple birth rates.

- **Does the specialist have experience in working with women with PCOS?** Since REs are highly specialized, they are able to provide women with PCOS a wider range of treatments, such as fertility drugs, advanced reproductive technologies, and surgical options.

- **Does the specialist have experience monitoring fertility drugs?** Once you decide to take fertility drugs, you want to be closely monitored to increase your chances of becoming pregnant and avoid complications.

- **Is the specialist qualified to do surgery?** If the fertility drugs do not work and you want to look into surgery, you want to make sure your fertility specialist is qualified to do such surgery.

- **What will treatment cost?** You want to know up front what to expect and how much everything will cost. Fertility treatments can be expensive and may not be covered by insurance. Also, make sure your fertility specialist's office has experience in working with insurance companies to ensure that they will make every effort possible to help you negotiate with your insurance company to possibly cover costs. (Sometimes, diagnostic tests such as blood work and ultrasounds arc covered by insurance.)

Methods to Monitor Ovulation

The first step in achieving pregnancy is to determine whether you are ovulating. Once you know that you are ovulating, you can plan intercourse to maximize your chances of becoming pregnant. Your physician may suggest several of the following methods to monitor your cycle to determine when ovulation is occurring.

Basal Body Temperature (BBT)

One way to determine whether you are ovulating is to check your *basal body temperature* (*BBT*), your body's temperature at rest. It should be taken at the same time each day—right before you get out of bed in the morning and after at least six hours of sleep.

Each day, your temperature should be charted on a special piece of graph paper. (Your physician can likely give you this form.) A cycle in which ovulation has occurred is characterized by a *biphasic temperature chart*. This means your temperature remains lower until the time of ovulation, when a rise occurs of about 0.2 degrees centigrade or more. The rise takes place abruptly soon *after* the egg is released. The rise is the result of increased progesterone levels. The temperature remains at the higher level until just before, or at the onset of, the next period. If you do not see a change in temperature, you are most likely not ovulating.

Anything unusual—a cold, a late night, drinking alcohol, or any stressful situation—can affect your temperature. Therefore, many women find it difficult to chart BBT. Even a half-hour delay in taking your temperature can reduce reliability.

Note that charting BBT can only indicate whether you have *already* ovulated. Therefore, it is not useful in timing intercourse to achieve pregnancy during that cycle. By the time your temperature has gone up, it is generally too late to conceive. However, some research indicates there is a slight temperature drop just prior to ovulation. The information is useful for knowing when you might try intercourse during the next cycle.

Still, since women with PCOS have irregular cycles with varying lengths, it can be impossible to predict when ovulation will occur the next month. Accordingly, charting BBT may be most helpful in determining whether your cycles are typically ovulatory or not. In addition, BBTs can be useful when planning to do multiple cycles of Clomid.

Examining Cervical Mucus

Another way to monitor cycles is to determine the color and consistency of cervical mucus. This may be done using either your fingers or toilet paper. In most women, cervical mucus varies from dry, to sticky, to creamy, to "egg-white" just before ovulation. Good cervical mucus at the time of ovulation is important to fertilization since it provides an optimal environment for sperm.

During a typical twenty-eight-day cycle, the consistency of cervical mucus should be as follows:

Days 1–5	Menses
Days 6–9	Dry, or little or no mucus
Days 10–12	Sticky, thick mucus, becoming less thick and whiter
Days 13–15 (most fertile time)	"Egg-white" mucus—thin, elastic, slippery, clear
Days 16–21	Sticky, thick mucus
Days 22–28	Dry mucus

When mucus is described as dry, this means you won't find much mucus to the touch. Sticky refers to having enough mucus to feel sticky between your fingers. The mucus may be creamy and feels somewhat like lotion when you rub your fingers together. The so-called "egg-white" mucus resembles raw egg whites. It can be either clear or streaked and stretches an inch or more. This represents a woman's most fertile time in the cycle. Since every woman is different, changes in cervical mucus can sometimes be hard to notice.

Ovulation Predictor Kits (OPK)

Ovulation predictor kits (OPKs) are sold over the counter and use urine to detect the LH surge that occurs just *before* the egg is released from the ovary. OPKs are especially useful if you are taking fertility medication. Since OPKs let you know right before the egg is released, you can use OPKs to plan intercourse.

There are many different brands of OPKs, including many name and generic brands. Most OPKs are simple to use. Urinate on the test stick, and about five to ten minutes later, it will determine whether you are having an LH surge by measuring the amount of LH in your urine. Usually, there are two lines on the test stick—the test line and the control line. If the test line is a lighter shade than the control line, you are not having an LH surge. If the test line is the same or a shade darker than the control line, an LH surge has been detected. Once the LH surge has been detected, you will most likely ovulate within the next twenty-four hours.

To ensure you catch the LH surge, you should begin testing a few days before you think you are going to ovulate. If you are taking fertility medication, talk to your doctor about when you should start testing, since fertility medication can change the length of your cycle or affect the test by causing a false positive.

Unfortunately, many women with PCOS cannot use OPKs since their LH levels might be high enough to give a false positive result. Since different OPKs measure LH at slightly different levels, you might want to try a few different brands when you are certain you are not ovulating to see if you get a false positive.

One product that might help women with PCOS determine their LH surge is a *fertility monitor.* It is similar to the traditional OPK in that it determines the LH surge by measuring the amount of LH in your urine. However, it uses actual numerical values instead of colored lines to record your LH level. This allows women with high levels of LH to still notice an LH surge by watching the numbers increase.

Diagnostic Tests to Monitor Ovulation

The most reliable way to determine if and when ovulation is occurring is to undergo a series of diagnostic tests performed by a physician. These tests are usually done in conjunction with charting BBT, noting cervical mucus, and/or using an OPK to determine the LH surge.

Transvaginal Ultrasound

As mentioned earlier, the transvaginal ultrasound may be used in diagnosing PCOS. The ultrasound is used to view your ovaries and to check the uterine lining. The doctor can examine the size of your ovaries to see exactly how many follicles are developing (which lets you know if you are at risk for multiple births) and how big they are. To be considered "ripe" and the optimum size for conception, follicles should measure about 18 to 20 millimeters in diameter. In addition, a uterine lining above 8 millimeters will sustain a pregnancy.

Seven-Day Post-Ovulation Progesterone Test

At about Day 21 in your cycle (or about seven days after you think you have ovulated), your doctor may suggest a *twenty-one-day post-ovulation progesterone test,* or *mid-luteal serum progesterone test.* This test will tell you if your egg was released from the ovary. If it was released, your progesterone levels should be significantly higher. Progesterone levels above 3 are consistent with ovulation, although ideally they should be above 10. If your progesterone levels are low, the egg most likely was not released.

Most often these tests are administered to women taking fertility medication. Some doctors suggest that women have an ultrasound, and a progesterone test during each cycle. Other physicians recommend only one or two of these tests during a cycle. Ultimately, the more closely your cycle is monitored, the better understanding you and your doctor will have about how to correct any problems.

Period or Pregnancy?

If you did indeed ovulate successfully, you should begin your period exactly fourteen days after the egg was released. If you do not start your period fourteen days after you ovulated, you might be pregnant. If this occurs, take a pregnancy test. If it comes back negative, wait a few days and retest. If it is still negative and you still have not started your period, call you doctor for further information. If it is determined that you did not ovulate, then your doctor may prescribe Provera or Prometrium to induce your period so you can start another cycle.

If you charted your basal body temperature, your temperature will stay high if you are pregnant. If your temperature starts dropping, then your period is impending.

Common Fertility Medications

The major benefit of taking fertility medication is that you may have a greater chance of becoming pregnant. These drugs work by stimulating egg production, encouraging ovulation, or stabilizing hormone levels which may be disrupting the fertilization process. Fortunately, a number of such medications are available for women with PCOS, but not every medication works for everyone. It may take trial and error to find one that works for you.

One of the risks of fertility medications is *ovarian hyperstimulation syndrome (OHSS),* a rare but serious condition in which the ovaries enlarge as a result of fertility medication and cause abdominal pain or discomfort, bloating, or nausea. More-severe forms of OHSS can involve blood clots, massive accumulation of fluid in the abdomen and pelvis (requiring surgical drainage), and damage to other organs such as the lungs, liver, and kidneys.

Clomiphene Citrate

Clomiphene citrate is the gold standard in fertility medication given to women with PCOS. It is also known by the brand names Clomid and Serophene. This drug, taken in pill form, works by causing the body to produce more FSH and LH, the hormones that promote egg growth. Once the brain senses increased estrogen levels, it signals the LH surge that results in ovulation.

While it may take several months to determine the right dosage of clomiphene citrate, the drug should not be taken for an extended period of time, even if it causes you to ovulate. It can actually have a negative effect on fertility by causing thick cervical mucus, which is hostile to sperm and inhibits fertilization. Additionally, taking the drug for longer than six months is unlikely to result in a pregnancy. If your doctor continues to recommend this treatment, it is reasonable to seek another opinion.

If a woman is going to ovulate on clomiphene citrate, she usually does so in the first three or four cycles. Some studies estimate that about 75 percent of women will ovulate on clomiphene citrate, with about 35 percent achieving pregnancy within six months.

Unfortunately, 20 to 30 percent of women with PCOS are "Clomid resistant." This means that they do not ovulate with clomiphene citrate, even at the maximum dosage. The drug does not affect insulin levels;

studies have shown that clomiphene citrate, when taken with an insulin sensitizer such as metformin, significantly increases ovulation but not pregnancy rate.

There are several potential side effects of clomiphene citrate. The most common side effects are hot flashes and vaginal dryness. There is also a slightly increased risk of conceiving twins or triplets. However, other potential side effects can be more serious. It's possible, but rare, to experience ovarian enlargement, even ovarian hyperstimulation. Other, rare side effects that need to be reported immediately to your physician include changes in vision and severe headaches. It is best to stop the medication immediately if you develop these symptoms.

Gonadotropins

Gonadotropins are drugs that stimulate the ovaries to produce and release eggs. The medications act by supplying a woman's body with an extra amount of the hormones FSH and LH, or FSH only—the hormones that start egg production.

The risks with gonadotropins include an increased chance of multiple births and ovarian hyperstimulation. The risk of multiple pregnancy is about 20 percent, with most of these being twins. The chance of ovarian hyperstimulation is less than 1 percent per cycle if gonadotropins are managed by competent doctors. Other possible side effects vary greatly from one woman to the next, but may include bloating, abdominal pain and nausea. Three common gonadotropins are listed below.

Human Chorionic Gonadotropin (hCG)

The drug *human chorionic gonadotropin (hCG)* is used with other fertility medications, including clomiphene citrate, FSH, and *human menopausal gonadotropin (hMG)*, to promote ovulation by triggering the LH surge. This drug, given by injection, is sold under the common brand names *Novarel, Ovidrel, Pregnyl,* and *Profasi.*

In some women with PCOS, a follicle successfully develops during the use of other fertility medications, but the egg is never released from the ovary. By performing a transvaginal ultrasound about the time ovulation should occur, the doctor can view the developing follicle. If the follicle appears "ripe" but the LH fails to surge and trigger the release of the egg, the doctor can give an injection of hCG. This should cause ovulation.

FSH Drugs

There are different types of FSH drugs available, depending on how they are prepared. Commonly prescribed include medications include *Gonal-f, Follistim,* and *Bravelle.* These drugs, given by daily injection, stimulate the ovaries to produce multiple eggs. Side effects include bloating and possible ovarian hyperstimulation.

Human Menopausal Gonadotropin (hMG)

An extract from the urine of menopausal women, human menopausal gonadotropin (hMG) contains LH and FSH, which stimulate ovulation. The drug is sold as *Menopur* and *Repronex*. This drug is given by injection, usually in the thigh or buttocks. A shot of hCG is then given later in the cycle to promote the release of the egg. Some research suggests that about 90 percent of women ovulate using hMG but only about 60 percent actually conceive. The risk of multiple births can be as high as 20 percent.

Several factors need to be considered before using hMG. Mood swings can be a side effect. Also, nearly 20 percent of women who take hMG may develop ovarian hyperstimulation if not monitored properly.

Insulin Sensitizers

Increasingly, insulin sensitizers, which were discussed in an earlier chapter, are considered the most effective method for treating infertility in women with PCOS since they bring insulin levels into balance. Many women with PCOS who did not previously ovulate while taking ovulation induction medications alone (including women who were Clomid resistant) will successfully ovulate while using insulin sensitizers. By using insulin sensitizers, such as Avandia and Glucophage, in conjunction with clomiphene citrate or another fertility medication, over half of women with PCOS will ovulate.

The use of insulin sensitizers is recommended when there is evidence of glucose intolerance. It is unclear if the use of insulin sensitizers are beneficial in women without glucose intolerance. Keep in mind that Clomid should be considered the first medication used in women with PCOS who are attempting pregnancy.

Ovarian Surgery

In some cases, ovarian surgery is an option for women with PCOS who wish to become pregnant. Surgery is not a cure for PCOS, but it can be performed to promote ovulation long enough for a woman to become pregnant. However, these surgeries have been performed in the past, and it is not clear whether they are any more effective than medications. Further, these surgeries are not recommended by the American College of Obstetrics and Gynecology (ACOG).

There are two types of ovarian surgery—ovarian drilling and wedge resection.

Of these two methods, *ovarian drilling* is the most common. It is an outpatient, laparoscopic procedure that uses a laser to pierce the thickened coat of the ovary. The surgeon uses the laser to penetrate the cysts on each ovary. Fluid is drained from the ovary, eliminating many of the cysts. In turn, the amount of androgens produced is lowered, causing a decrease in LH.

About 80 percent of women undergoing this procedure will ovulate, and about 30 to 40 percent will become pregnant. Women at or close to ideal body weight usually have better results after surgery than those who are overweight. Risks involved with ovarian drilling include the normal risks of surgery, such as bleeding and infection. Although it is a noninvasive procedure, ovarian drilling still carries the risks of possible adhesions and excessive destruction of the ovary, which could result in ovarian failure.

Wedge resection, a major procedure in which cysts are surgically removed from the ovaries, was used successfully in the management of women with PCOS prior to the availability of antiestrogens in the 1960s. It resulted in a high rate of ovulation but was followed by significant formation of adhesions that prevented pregnancy a few months after the procedure was performed. The procedure is seldom used today.

Advanced Reproductive Technologies

Some women with PCOS who are not successful at getting pregnant using traditional methods of treating PCOS-related infertility turn to *advanced reproductive technologies (ARTs).* These procedures are carried out daily in clinics across the nation.

The success rates of ARTs are quite variable. Success depends on many factors, including age, other medical or reproductive problems (both male and female), the experience of the medical team and clinic, the quality of the eggs and sperm, the number of embryos implanted, and the number of cycles attempted, to name just a few.

If you are interested in finding out more about ARTs, you should consult a reproductive endocrinologist or other fertility specialist for an individual evaluation. He/she can assess your specific medical situation and your chances of success using ARTs.

Intrauterine Insemination (IUI)

For an *intrauterine insemination (IUI)* procedure, egg production is stimulated through the use of fertility medications and monitored closely by the attending physician. As soon as it is clear that the woman is successfully ovulating, sperm from her partner or donor is washed and deposited directly into the uterus. (Washing the sperm separates sperm cells from semen, helping to get rid of dead or slow-moving sperm as well as additional chemicals that may impair fertilization.) The goal is to concentrate the number of healthy, moving sperm in the washed specimen, shortening the distance to the ovary by bypassing the vagina, cervix, and most of the uterus.

In Vitro Fertilization (IVF)

In vitro fertilization (IVF) involves retrieving the eggs from a woman's ovaries and fertilizing them with sperm in a laboratory. Once fertilization occurs, the fertilized egg or eggs are returned to the uterus for implantation.

IVF is currently considered safer than using injectable gonadotropins alone because of the decreased risk of higher-number multiple births; parents of higher-order multiples, such as triplets, quadruplets, or quintuplets face challenges in raising them.

Several studies have suggested that it may be more effective if you go directly to IVF if you fail to get pregnant on Clomid. However, injectable gonadotropins are safe and do have a role in the treatment of infertility when used by an experienced physician.

Intracytoplasmic Sperm Injection

In *intracytoplasmic sperm injection*, a single sperm is injected into an egg through a very tiny needle. This procedure is performed under a microscope in an IV laboratory. Three to five days later, depending on the quality of the embryo, the resulting embryo is transferred into the uterus.

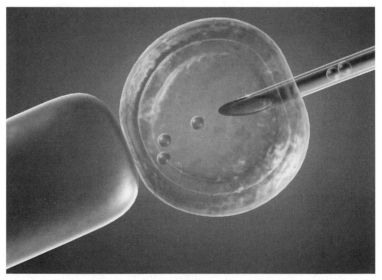

An intracytoplasmic sperm injection, shown above, is a laboratory procedure, in which sperm is injected into an egg. If healthy, the embryo is transferred to the uterus days later.

Donor Eggs

Egg donation, also referred to as oocyte donation, makes pregnancy possible for women who might not otherwise be able to get pregnant using their own eggs. The donor eggs are fertilized in the lab with the sperm from a mate or donor. Once fertilized, the eggs are placed inside the uterus. Although the woman is not the genetic mother, she will carry the baby and give birth.

If Conception Does Not Occur

Although many women with PCOS can get pregnant and successfully carry a pregnancy to term, not all women with PCOS can do so. Other factors may play a role in their not being able to conceive, and advanced reproductive technology does not work for all women. After months and sometimes years of treatment, both the medical and emotional costs can be high. As such, many couples are faced with making difficult choices. They may decide to remain child-free or choose to bring a child into their family through surrogacy, adoption, or foster care.

Other Fertility Problems

Sometimes women with PCOS can also have other fertility problems such as endometriosis, fallopian tube blockage, uterine abnormalities, and excess prolactin (the hormone that stimulates milk production). It is important to rule such problems before any fertility treatments are started. This may include having a *hysterosalpingogram (HSG),* in which dye is injected into the uterus and fallopian tubes and X-rays are taken to look for abnormalities or blockages. Or perhaps male factors such as inadequate sperm may be a problem. A test of the male's sperm may be called for.

Still, other times, there may be no apparent reason for a woman's infertility. This can occur when everything seems to be working—the cycle is normal, ovulating is occurring, the eggs are of good quality, the amount of sperm is adequate, and the cervical mucus is good. But still there is no pregnancy. If this happens to you, talk to your physician about what to do next. He or she may order more-extensive testing or recommend a break from fertility treatments to give your body and your mind a well-deserved rest.

Secondary infertility refers to problems in conceiving after having no problems with a first pregnancy. Some women with PCOS who had little or no difficulty conceiving their first child may have tremendous difficulty getting pregnant a second time. This could be due to several factors, including increased age, continued changes in hormone levels, increased weight gain, or worsening of PCOS.

6

Maintaining a Pregnancy

Women with PCOS have a miscarriage rate that is 20 to 40 percent higher than that of women without PCOS. In fact, some studies of couples seeking to become pregnant have shown that as many as 50 percent of all pregnancies are lost, with the majority of them being lost early and not clinically recognized. Infertile couples appear to have a slightly higher miscarriage rate than fertile couples. Many factors can contribute to miscarriages both for women who have PCOS and for those who don't. These factors include:

- Age (After age thirty-five, as age increases so do miscarriage rates.)
- Uterine cavity abnormalities
- Chromosomal abnormalities
- Blood-clotting disorders
- Autoimmune disorders (such as lupus, arthritis, and thyroid disease)

The more risk factors you have, the higher your risk of a miscarriage. Many endocrinologists now believe that pregnancy in women with PCOS carries elevated risks of miscarriage, diabetes, and other problems. Accordingly, it is important to see your health-care provider as soon as possible after you discover that you are pregnant.

Most pregnant women with PCOS can see a regular OB/GYN or midwife for their prenatal care. Some women, especially those with diabetes or hypertension, may be referred to an OB/GYN or a fetal medicine specialist, who specializes in high-risk obstetrical care. The health-care provider may use any of several methods to help you maintain your pregnancy.

Supplementing Progesterone

Women with PCOS are often prescribed progesterone supplements if their progesterone levels are too low to sustain a pregnancy. During the first trimester of pregnancy, the mother's body produces the hormone progesterone to keep the uterus in good condition to support the pregnancy. After the first trimester, the placenta takes over producing the progesterone. If a woman is not producing enough progesterone during the early part of pregnancy, a miscarriage will occur.

Insulin Sensitizers

There is some controversy over whether it is safe to continue taking insulin sensitizers after conception.

Symptoms of Gestational Diabetes

- Increased thirst
- Increased urination
- Weight loss in spite of increased appetite
- Fatigue
- Nausea
- Vomiting
- Infections (including bladder, vaginal, skin)
- Blurred vision

Some studies have indicated that these drugs lessen the likelihood of miscarriage; other studies indicate they may increase the frequency of miscarriage. This is a matter you should discuss with your OB/GYN physician.

Pregnancy-Related Concerns

According to some surveys, women with PCOS face a greater risk of complications during pregnancy. Specifically, they face a greater risk of gestational diabetes. There may some increase in the risk for *preeclampsia* and for *eclampsia*, both of which are discussed in this section.

Cysts

Because women with PCOS are prone to developing cysts, it is not uncommon to have an ovarian cyst during pregnancy. Generally, the cyst will either dissipate on its own or rupture. A ruptured cyst can be painful, but it is not generally harmful to the mother or child. However, sometimes the cyst can twist the ovary, requiring emergency surgery. Still, a cyst may impede delivery and may require a cesarean section.

A cyst that is less than 10 millimeters in size does not need to be removed; however, those that are 20 millimeters or larger and persistent need to be evaluated.

Gestational Diabetes

Women with PCOS may be more likely to develop *gestational diabetes*, or glucose intolerance, during pregnancy. Gestational diabetes is usually discovered during the twenty-fourth to twenty-eighth weeks of pregnancy with routine screening. The symptoms are usually mild and not life-threatening to a pregnant woman; however, the increased maternal fasting glucose levels are associated with an increased rate of fetal or newborn deaths. Maintaining control of blood glucose levels significantly reduces the risk to the baby.

The risk factors for gestational diabetes are a maternal age of thirty-five or older, a family history of diabetes, obesity, and a birth weight over nine pounds in a previous infant.

Women with PCOS who are overweight or who have gestational diabetes may have large fetuses, a condition known as *macrosomia*. This can sometimes result in difficult births and cesarean sections. The infant born to a woman with gestational diabetes may have an increased birth weight, have low blood glucose levels during the early newborn period, and be jaundiced.

The goals of treatment are to maintain blood glucose levels within normal limits for the duration of the pregnancy and to ensure the well-being of the fetus. Fetal monitoring to assess fetal size and well-being may include ultrasound exams. Diet management provides adequate calories and nutrients, and control of blood glucose levels. Nutritional counseling by a registered dietician is recommended. Exercise can also be very effective in controlling gestational diabetes.

If dietary management does not control blood glucose levels within the recommended range, your doctor may consider insulin therapy. Blood glucose self-monitoring is required for effective treatment with insulin.

High blood glucose levels often resolve after pregnancy. However, women with gestational diabetes should be followed postpartum and at regular intervals for early detection of diabetes. Up to 30 to 40 percent of women with gestational diabetes develop overt diabetes within five to ten years after delivery. The risk may be higher if the woman is considered obese. Many doctors recommend screening early in the pregnancy if you have risk factors for gestational diabetes.

Preeclampsia and Eclampsia

There are some indications that women with PCOS may be more likely to develop a type of high

Signs and Symptoms of Preeclampsia

- Edema (swelling of the hands and face, or severe swelling anywhere on the body)
- Unintentional weight gain in excess of two pounds per week (Gain may be sudden over one to two days.)
- Headaches that don't go away with treatment
- Decreased urine output
- Nausea and vomiting
- High or elevated blood pressure
- Agitation
- Chest or upper abdominal pain
- Proteinuria (protein in urine)
- Thrombocytopenia (a decrease in the number of circulating blood platelets)

blood pressure known as *preeclampsia.* It's also called *pregnancy-induced hypertension,* or *toxemia.* If left untreated, preeclampsia can develop into *eclampsia,* a full-blown form of the illness, marked by seizures and/or coma. Eclampsia is a serious problem and is the leading cause of maternal death. However, if proper medical care is given, it is very unusual for eclampsia to develop.

The exact cause of preeclampsia has not been identified. Numerous theories about the cause exist, including genetic, low-protein intake, vascular (blood vessel), and neurological factors. None of the theories have yet been proven. Preeclampsia occurs in approximately 5 percent of all pregnancies. Increased risk is associated with first pregnancies, teenage mothers, mothers more than forty years old, African-American women, multiple pregnancies, and women with a history of diabetes, hypertension, or kidney disease. Because many women with PCOS are insulin resistant and may have hypertension, the risks are greater.

Although there are currently no known ways to prevent these complications, it is important for all pregnant women to obtain early and ongoing prenatal care. This allows for the early recognition and treatment of conditions such as preeclampsia. "I developed preeclampsia three and a half weeks before my due date. I had slowly started having problems, and one day my blood pressure shot through the roof. My daughter was born later that night. It was incredibly frightening," Anna, age twenty-three, remembered.

The best treatment for preeclampsia is bed rest and delivery as soon as possible for the baby. Patients are usually hospitalized, but occasionally they may be managed on an outpatient basis with careful monitoring of blood pressure and weight and with urine checks for protein. Optimally, the condition may be managed until a delivery after thirty-six weeks of pregnancy.

In severe cases of preeclampsia with the pregnancy beyond twenty-eight weeks, delivery is the treatment of choice. For pregnancies less than twenty-four weeks, the induction of labor is recommended, although the likelihood of a viable fetus is minimal. Prolonging such pregnancies has shown to result in maternal complications as well as infant death in approximately 87 percent of cases. Pregnancies between twenty-four and twenty-eight weeks present a "gray zone," and conservative management may be attempted, with monitoring for maternal and fetal complications. Because there are not clear guidelines for less-severe cases of preeclampsia, frequent follow-up of fetus and mother is necessary, as is continued revision of the treatment plan.

Maternal deaths caused by preeclampsia are rare in the United States. Fetal or perinatal deaths do sometimes occur, yet the chance of death decreases as the fetus matures. The risk of recurrent preeclampsia in subsequent pregnancies is approximately 33 percent. Preeclampsia does not appear to lead to chronic high blood pressure.

Breast-Feeding Concerns

Many women with PCOS are successful when it comes to breast-feeding; others experience the same difficulties as women in the general population. Some research indicates there may be problems with milk supply in mothers with PCOS. Pregnant women who wish to breast-feed should find a lactation consultant prior to delivery in case one is needed.

7

Long-Term Risks of PCOS

S usan, age forty, had experienced PCOS-related symptoms for as long as she could remember. In fact, when she was in her mid-twenties, her doctor suspected that she had PCOS and told her so. Even though her symptoms could sometimes be annoying, they never really bothered her too much. Susan was a successful businesswoman. She had just gotten married, and she and her new husband had decided that they did not want to have children. Both wanted to remain career focused. As a result, Susan really wasn't concerned about her irregular periods. She actually thought of herself as rather lucky, not having to worry about it every month.

As she was looking through the newspaper one Sunday afternoon, she noticed an article about PCOS in the health section. The article mentioned something about research that linked PCOS to heart disease and diabetes. Susan was surprised to read this and wondered if she should see a doctor about her suspected PCOS.

Type 2 Diabetes

It is estimated that at least half of all women with PCOS have detectable insulin resistance. All women with PCOS who have insulin resistance are at serious risk for developing Type 2 diabetes at some point in their lives. In fact, everyone who develops Type 2 diabetes starts off having insulin resistance first. The problems caused by insulin resistance just get worse until the body is no longer able to utilize the insulin at all. This results in diabetes.

Unfortunately, there are often few or no symptoms to alert you that this is happening. Women with PCOS should have their blood tested regularly for insulin resistance and diabetes. You are at even higher risk for developing Type 2 diabetes if you:

- Weigh 20 percent more than your ideal body weight
- Have high blood pressure
- Have low HDL cholesterol levels (under 35 mg/dL)
- Have high triglyceride levels (over 200 mg/dL)
- Have a close relative with diabetes
- Are from a high-risk ethnic group
- Are over age forty
- Have delivered a baby weighing over nine pounds
- Have a history of gestational diabetes

Types of Diabetes

Diabetes is a metabolic disease characterized by high blood sugar levels, which result from defects in insulin secretion. In the United States, nearly 24 million people, or 8 percent of the population, have diabetes. It is the seventh leading cause of death.

Type 1 diabetes usually develops during childhood or adolescence and occurs when the body does not produce insulin, the hormone needed to convert sugars into energy.

Type 2 diabetes is the result of the body not producing enough insulin or the body's cells not responding to it. Type 2 diabetes can develop in youth as well as in adults.

Gestational diabetes occurs in pregnant women who have not previously had diabetes but whose blood sugars become elevated during pregnancy. Hormones block the mother's insulin, causing a buildup of insulin, or insulin resistance.

Type 2 diabetes is a chronic condition that has no cure. In people with Type 2 diabetes, glucose builds up in the blood. However, with proper treatment, your blood sugar levels can return to normal again. A "normal" sugar level does not mean you are cured and no longer have diabetes. Instead, it shows that your treatment plan is effective and that you are doing a good job of controlling your diabetes.

The goal for treating diabetes is to lower your blood sugar (glucose) levels and improve your body's use of insulin. This can be achieved in a variety of ways, including meal planning, exercise, weight loss, and taking medications.

Since your body breaks down food into glucose, your blood sugar level rises when you eat. You want to exercise good meal planning that slows down this rise in sugar. You want to try to choose foods that are low in fat, have protein, and contain only moderate amounts of carbohydrates. Many nutritionists and dieticians specialize in helping people who either have diabetes or are at risk for developing diabetes make better meal choices in order to successfully manage their blood sugar levels.

Being active also helps your body more efficiently process glucose and utilize insulin. If you don't currently exercise regularly, you might want to become more active. Ideally, you should be active on most days of the week for a total of thirty minutes per day, which can be broken down into shorter five-to ten-minute sessions. If you are not used to exercising regularly, start slow. Even a five-minute walk is good. However, before you start any exercise plan, you should always talk to your health-care provider first.

Losing weight is another big part of managing diabetes. It will help you utilize insulin better. Ask your health-care provider how much weight you should lose. Also find out the most effective way for you to lose weight. Sometimes, losing just ten or twenty pounds is enough to better control your diabetes.

As explained in previous chapters, physicians often prescribe insulin sensitizers to help control diabetes and bring glucose and insulin levels back to normal. However, taking these medications does not replace the need for healthful habits, including eating well and exercising.

If not successfully managed, diabetes can lead to serious medical complications, including heart disease, stroke, eye and kidney problems, and problems involving the blood vessels, nerves, and feet. It is important to mention that these treatment methods for controlling Type 2 diabetes can also be effective in managing insulin resistance. Women with PCOS who maintain appropriate blood glucose and insulin levels can significantly lessen the risk of developing diabetes while also minimizing some of the other effects of PCOS.

Cardiovascular Disease

Researchers are beginning to understand the connection between PCOS, heart disease, and stroke. In the past few years, numerous studies have found that women with PCOS have a seven times greater risk of developing cardiovascular disease than women without PCOS. This is probably due to the fact that women with PCOS also tend to have more of the risk factors associated with cardiovascular disease.

The major risk factors for heart disease and stroke are:

- Cigarette/tobacco smoking
- High blood cholesterol (over 200 mg/dL)
- High blood pressure (over 120/80 mm/Hg)
- Physical inactivity

- Heredity (family history of cardiovascular disease, especially if early onset)
- Male gender
- Increasing age
- Other contributing factors such as diabetes, obesity, and stress

Women with PCOS have a greater tendency to be overweight or obese and have higher levels of cholesterol and blood pressure. The risk for heart disease increases for women with PCOS who smoke, have a family history of cardiovascular disease, are under a lot of stress, or are physically inactive. The bottom line is, the more risk factors you have, the greater chance you will develop cardiovascular disease, which could result in a heart attack or stroke.

To lower your risk for heart disease and stroke, it is important to seek treatment. By directly treating PCOS, one might be able to bring hormone levels into a normal range, minimizing or eliminating the symptoms and effects of PCOS, including high cholesterol and insulin levels. In some cases, there may be a need for additional medications such as those for high cholesterol and high blood pressure.

Also, it is important to make appropriate lifestyle changes as part of your treatment plan to prevent heart disease. Being overweight and physically inactive can significantly increase your chance of developing heart disease. Talk to your physician about safe and effective ways to lose weight and increase your

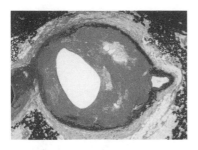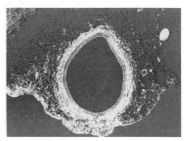

In the blocked artery, on the left, plaque buildup obstructs the flow of blood. The white area in the center is the only portion of the artery not blocked. On the right, the normal artery is open, able to transport oxygenated blood away from the heart to other parts of the body. *Photo courtesy of Custom Medical Stock.*

exercise. It is important that any weight loss plan you choose takes into consideration your PCOS.

Endometrial Hyperplasia

Since most women with PCOS do not have normal menstrual cycles, the uterine lining is not shed and replaced each month. As a result, old cells continue to build up within the uterus. The more time that passes without a period, the more buildup occurs. Sometimes, this buildup can cause *endometrial hyperplasia*, an overgrowth of the endometrium, which can be a precursor to cancer. There are several degrees of hyperplasia. *Simple hyperplasia* holds the least risk for developing endometrial cancer, whereas hyperplasia with *atypia* (a pathological term for the presence of abnormal, precancerous cells) holds a much higher risk—25 to 30 percent or greater.

The longer you go without a period, the greater your chance of developing endometrial hyperplasia

Metabolic Syndrome

Women with PCOS are at greater risk for having metabolic syndrome, which increases the risk for heart attack and stroke. Anyone with three or more of the abnormalities listed in the criteria below is considered as having the syndrome.

1. *High Fasting Blood Glucose.* This means blood sugar, or glucose, levels are high when tested after fasting, but are not high enough to be classified as diabetes.

2. *Abdominal obesity.* The belly fat, or "central obesity," is a key risk factor.

3. *Low HDL cholesterol.* The high-density lipoprotein cholesterol, or HDL, is commonly known as the "good" cholesterol.

4. *High triglycerides.* Triglycerides are a form of fat the body uses for energy. The medical term for high triglycerides is *hypertriglyceridemia*.

5. *High blood pressure.* High blood pressure occurs when the force of blood flowing through the artery walls is too high. High blood pressure is also referred to as *hypertension*.

This criteria for metabolic syndrome is the one most commonly accepted by medical professionals. It was developed by the National Cholesterol Education Program of the National Heart, Lung, and Blood Institute.

and perhaps cancer. This is why it is important to seek medical help if you have abnormal or absent periods. Many women with PCOS think that if they are not trying to become pregnant, it is okay to miss periods. Most physicians do not advise women to go more than a few months without a period.

Cancer

If left untreated, endometrial hyperplasia can develop into cancer of the uterus or the endometrium. If your physician is concerned that your uterine lining is too thick, placing you at risk for developing endometrial or uterine cancer, he/she might suggest that you have a *dilation and curettage (D & C),* in which the cervix is opened and the lining of the uterus is surgically scraped out. After the procedure is completed, most women experience bleeding and abdominal cramping for a few days. Your physician may also order an *endometrial biopsy* so that a portion of the endometrial tissue can be examined in the lab. Both D & Cs and endometrial biopsies are outpatient procedures done under local anesthesia.

Women with a family history of cancer or increased levels of estrogen face an even greater risk of developing endometrial cancer. The primary way to reduce your risk for developing endometrial or uterine cancer is to make sure that you see your health-care provider for a complete gynecological exam each year. He/she can help you maintain regular periods, which should also reduce your risk.

8

Hope for the Future

S ince childhood, Brianna, age thirty-six, had always wanted to work in the medical field. She earned a degree in nursing and loved working as a nurse in a busy pediatrician's office. Because of her medical background, Brianna immediately wanted to know what research was being conducted to learn more about PCOS. Fortunately, her doctor taught classes at the local medical school, so he put her in touch with a researcher who was conducting a study about diet and PCOS.

Brianna signed up for the study right away. It was a simple research study that lasted only a few months. She was asked to keep a log of everything she ate and to answer a number of questions about her nutrition and exercise habits and her PCOS symptoms. Brianna really felt good about being part of a study that might help other women with PCOS. Now she volunteers occasionally at the medical school, educating other women about participating in studies.

Research Studies and Clinical Trials

Research is ongoing to find out more about PCOS. Women with PCOS have the opportunity to be involved in this cutting-edge research by participating in research studies and clinical trials. A basic *research study* gathers and interprets information. It usually involves participants answering questions via a survey or interview.

A *clinical trial* is a well-planned research study that involves the administration of a test treatment, such as a drug. In most cases, those who receive treatment are compared to a *control group* that does not receive the treatment. Any differences between these two groups are noted and perhaps studied further.

To make the studies more effective, clinical trials are often masked, or blinded. That is, some information is withheld from either the study participant and/or the physician conducting the study. Clinical trials can be single-blind, double-blind, or triple-blind.

In *single-blind trials*, usually the study physician knows whether the study participant is assigned to the treatment or control group, but this information is not given to the participant. In *double-blind trials*, neither the study physician nor the study participant knows to which group the participant has been assigned.

Finally, in *triple-blind trials*, no one, not even the researchers responsible for the trial, knows to which group each participant belongs. These are rare with medication trials since a monitoring committee will ordinarily review the data periodically to ensure there is no harm to the participants.

Once the trial is completed, all the information is released. However, it may be months (even years for some larger trials) before the information is available to local investigators and participants.

Participation in a Clinical Trial

If you are interested in participating in a research study or clinical trial, first ask your physician about any research that is being conducted in your area. You can also contact your local medical school or teaching hospital (usually a hospital that is affiliated with a medical school or university). Most often, the endocrinology or gynecology department is interested in conducting research on PCOS.

In addition, you can also find out about national studies by contacting the National Institutes of Health in Bethesda, Maryland. The Polycystic Ovarian Syndrome Association (PCOSA) keeps an up-to-date list of current research opportunities on its Web site. Sometimes, a study requires that you live close to the research center. This is especially true of clinical trials. However, some research studies are just trying to gather information, and the researchers will interview women nationwide. They will simply have you complete a survey or a telephone interview.

Before participating in a clinical trial, however, you should ask the following questions:

- **Who is responsible for conducting the clinical trial?** Make sure both the researcher and the study site are reputable and have a good history of conducting clinical trials.

- **What are the participant requirements?** Many studies are specific regarding which types of people they need. For instance, they might be looking for women age eighteen to twenty-five who are not interested in becoming pregnant over the next few months. Make sure you fit the requirements.

- **What commitment must be made?** Sometimes, participating in a clinical trial means many trips to the study site, while other times, it may require a single visit. Make sure you can fulfill the commitment you make. Also, make sure you ask about such requirements as blood work, examinations, and interviews.

- **What is the compensation?** Most clinical trials offer payment or some type of compensation. Usually, the more time-intensive a trial is, the greater the compensation. Also, all associated medications, lab tests, and physical examinations should be provided at no cost to you.

- **Is the trial masked?** Will you be told whether you have been assigned to the treatment group or control group? If medication is involved, the control group is usually given a placebo so that they will not know they are not actually taking the medication. Most likely, you will not know to which group you have been assigned until after the study is completed.

- **What is the purpose of the clinical trial?**
  What is this clinical trial trying to accomplish? For example, is it to study the effectiveness of a new medication? To try new methods to treat PCOS-related infertility? To determine how certain foods affect PCOS? To determine whether PCOS runs in families? Make sure you are comfortable with the goals of the trial.

- **Will I be asked to sign a consent form?** You should *always* be asked to sign a consent form before you participate in a clinical trial. This form should explain all the details of the clinical trial and tell you exactly what you should expect. You should be given the opportunity to have all your questions about the trial answered. If you have any unanswered questions or are unclear about any aspect of the study, do not sign the consent form until you get the information that you need.

- **Will I learn the results of the study?** It is important to know what is going to happen after the clinical trial is completed. Will you find out if you were a part of the treatment or control group? Will you be given the opportunity to receive the treatment if it is found to be effective? Where will the results be published? How will study participants hear about the results?

Research on PCOS

Research studies and clinical trials addressing PCOS continue. Some of the major areas being studied are:

- Further information about the connection between PCOS and insulin resistance
- PCOS and genetics
- New medications to manage PCOS
- Medications and treatments that aid in fertility for women with PCOS
- The influence of PCOS on the risk of developing heart disease
- How PCOS affects moods
- The impact of diet and exercise on PCOS
- PCOS in adolescents

A Final Note

Unfortunately, there is still a lot we don't know about PCOS. The good news is, we are learning more and more each day. As a result, there are already many more treatment options available for women than there were a decade ago. As time goes by and more research is conducted, there is a good chance that PCOS will be even better controlled and perhaps one day even cured.

Resources

American Academy of Dermatology
P.O. Box 4014
Schaumburg, IL 60168-4014
(866) 503-SKIN (7546)
www.aad.org

American Association of Naturopathic Physicians
4435 Wisconsin Avenue, NW
Suite 403
Washington, DC 20016
(866) 538-2267
www.naturopathic.org

American Cancer Society (ACS)
1955 Clifton Road
Atlanta, GA 30329
(800) 227-2345
www.cancer.org

American College of Obstetricians and Gynecologists (ACOG)
409 12th Street, SW
P.O. Box 96920

Washington, DC 20090-6920
(202) 638-5577
www.acog.org

American Diabetes Association
1701 North Beauregard Street
Alexandria, VA 22311
(800) DIABETES (342-2383)
www.diabetes.org

American Fertility Association (AFA)
305 Madison Avenue
Suite 449
New York, NY 10165
(888) 917-3777
www.theafa.org

American Hair Loss Council (AHLC)
30 South Main
Shenandoah, PA 17976
www.ahlc.org

American Headache Society
19 Mantua Road
Mount Royal, NJ 08061
(856) 423-0082
www.AmericanHeadacheSociety.org

American Heart Association
7272 Greenville Avenue
Dallas, TX 75231
(800) 242-8721
www.americanheart.org

American Society for Reproductive Medicine (ASRM)
(Formerly the American Fertility Society)

1209 Montgomery Highway
Birmingham, AL 35216-2809
(205) 978-5000
www.asrm.org

CenterWatch, Inc.
100 North Washington Street
Suite 301
Boston, MA 02114
(617) 948-5100
www.centerwatch.com

The Endocrine Society
8401 Connecticut Avenue
Suite 900
Chevy Chase, MD 20815
(888) 363-6274
www.endo-society.org

Fertility Research Foundation (FRF)
877 Park Avenue
New York, NY 10021
(888) 439-2999
www.frfbaby.com

International Council on Infertility Information Dissemination (INCIID)
P.O. Box 6836
Arlington, VA 22206
(703) 379-9178
www.inciid.org

The International Foundation for Research and Education (iFred)
P.O. Box 17598
Baltimore, MD   21297-1598
(800) 422-HOPE (4673)
www.ifred.org

National Cancer Institute
6116 Executive Boulevard
Room 3036A

Bethesda, MD 20892-8322
(800) 4-CANCER (422-6237)
www.nci.nih.gov

National Center for Complementary and Alternative Medicine
NCCAM Clearinghouse
P.O. Box 7923
Gaithersburg, MD 20898
(888) 644-6226
TTY/TDY: (866) 464-3615
Fax: (866) 464-3616
www.nccam.nih.gov

National Diabetes Information Clearinghouse (NDIC)
1 Information Way
Bethesda, MD 20892-3560
(800) 860–8747
www.diabetes.niddk.nih.gov

National Women's Health Resource Center (NWHRC)
157 Broad Street
Suite 106
Red Bank, NJ 07701
(877) 986-9472
www.healthywoman.org

Polycystic Ovarian Syndrome Association (PCOSA)
P.O. Box 3403
Englewood, CO 80111
www.pcosupport.org

RESOLVE
The National Infertility Association
1760 Old Meadow Road
Suite 500
McLean, VA 22102
(703) 556-7172
www.resolve.org

Society for Clinical and Medical Hair Removal
2810 Crossroads Drive
Suite 3800
Madison, WI 53718
(608) 443-2470
www.scmhr.org

Soulcysters
c/o Digital Media Group
836 La Cienega Boulevard #246
West Hollywood, CA 90069
www.soulcysters.com

Glossary

Acne: Inflammatory disease that affects the sebaceous glands of the skin.

Alopecia: Hair loss or baldness.

Amenorrhea: Absence of menstrual periods.

Androgens: Male hormones responsible for secondary male characteristics, including hair growth, voice change, and muscle development.

Anovulation: Absence of ovulation, or monthly release of an egg, from the ovary.

Antiandrogen: Blocks the effects of androgens, normally by blocking the receptor sites.

Basal body temperature (BBT): Temperature of the body taken at rest. Theoretically, BBT rises after ovulation has occurred.

Biopsy: Removal of a sample of tissue for diagnostic examination.

Blood sugar: Level of glucose present in the bloodstream, used by the brain and muscles as energy.

Carbohydrate: Basic component of food composed of chains of sugars. Short chains are referred to as simple carbohydrates and include table sugar, honey, maple syrup, and fruit sugars. These simple sugars are converted by the body into glucose, which affects insulin levels. Long chains are called

130

complex carbohydrates and include those found in starchy foods such as breads, cereals, potatoes, fruits, and vegetables. These are broken down by the body into glucose more slowly and are either used for immediate energy or are stored by the body for later use.

Cervical mucus: Lubricant secreted by the cervix and vaginal walls. Cervical mucus usually changes consistency around the time of ovulation to encourage fertilization.

Cervix: Lowermost part of the uterus.

Cholesterol: Waxy substance found in animal fat. In excess, it lines the artery walls, reducing blood flow.

Clomiphene citrate: Drug most commonly used to induce ovulation. Popular brand name is Clomid.

Corpus luteum: Yellow-colored mass in the ovary formed when the ovarian follicle has matured and released its egg. Responsible for secreting estrogen and progesterone. If fertilization occurs, the corpus luteum sustains the pregnancy until the placenta is formed and takes over.

Cyst: Abnormal sac usually containing fluid or solid material.

DHEAS: An androgen secreted by the adrenal gland.

Diabetes: Disease that affects blood sugar and causes inappropriate levels of insulin. Type 1, or juvenile diabetes, causes a decreased production of insulin. Type 2, or adult-onset diabetes, causes resistance to insulin.

Dilation and curettage (D&C): Dilating the cervix and scraping out the endometrium (lining) of the uterus.

Dysmenorrhea: Very painful menstruation.

Ectopic pregnancy: Pregnancy that occurs when the fertilized egg implants outside the uterus, usually in the fallopian tube.

Endocrine: Pertaining to the body's system that produces hormones.

Endocrinologist: Physician who specializes in the diagnosis and treatment of diseases affecting the endocrine system.

Endometrial hyperplasia: Overgrowth of uterine lining (endometriosis), usually due to the influence of prolonged estrogen exposure.

Endometrium: Lining of the uterus.

Estradiol: Most active, naturally occurring estrogen, a female hormone.

Estrogen: Female sex hormone produced by the ovaries and adrenal gland that causes the development of the female characteristics and also plays a role in menstruation and pregnancy.

Fallopian tubes: Structures located between the uterus and ovaries that are responsible for transporting the egg.

Fertilization: Joining of the sperm and egg, the first step in forming an embryo.

Follicle: Receptacle within the ovary that contains the immature egg.

Follicle-stimulating hormone (FSH): Causes the maturation and release of an egg each month.

Galactorrhea: Milk production and release from the breasts unrelated to nursing.

Gamete intro fallopian transfer (GIFT): Surgical procedure by which sperm and egg are injected directly into a woman's fallopian tubes.

Glucose: Simple sugar molecule, the principal sugar that circulates in the bloodstream.

Gonadotropin: Substance having a stimulating effect on the ovaries or testes.

Gonadotropin-releasing hormones (GnRH): Substances released from the hypothalamus, the part of the brain that controls reproduction, to stimulate the pituitary to produce gonadotropins, which, in turn, stimulate the ovaries to produce sex steroids.

High blood pressure: Condition in which the heart pumps blood through the circulatory system at a pressure greater than normal.

Hirsutism: Excessive hair growth.

Human chorionic gonadotropin (hCG): Substance derived from the urine of pregnant women. This is what home pregnancy tests detect to confirm pregnancy.

Human menopausal gonadotropin (hMG): Extract from the urine of menopausal women that contains LH and FSH. Used to stimulate ovulation.

Hyperandrogenism: Condition in which a woman has high levels of male sex hormones (androgens).

Hyperprolactinemia: Excess production of prolactin, the hormone responsible for promoting milk production.

Hypothalamus: Part of the brain responsible for maintaining body temperature, sleep, and hunger. Controls the hormones that regulate menstruation.

Hysterosalpingogram (HSG): Diagnostic test during which dye is injected into the uterus and fallopian tubes. X-rays are then taken to determine if there are any abnormalities or blockages.

Ideal body weight: Weight goal of an individual. It takes into consideration body type, muscle mass, and bone structure.

Insulin: Hormone produced by the pancreas. Insulin converts glucose from the bloodstream into glycogen, which is stored in muscle tissue and the liver.

Insulin resistance: Failure of the body to respond properly to the insulin produced by the pancreas. Related to diabetes.

Insulin sensitizers: Group of medications originally used to treat Type 2 diabetes but now sometimes used to alleviate many PCOS-related symptoms by helping to correct insulin resistance.

Intrauterine insemination (IUI): When a very thin, flexible catheter is threaded through the cervix and washed sperm is injected into the uterus.

In vitro fertilization (IVF): Uniting the sperm and egg outside the body under laboratory conditions. The fertilized egg is then returned to the woman's body in the hope that it will implant.

Laparoscope: Fiber-optic scope inserted through the navel to view the reproductive organs.

Luteinizing hormone (LH): Hormone that facilitates the conversion of the follicle into the corpus luteum.

Menarche: Very first occurrence of menstruation.

Menopause: When menstruation has stopped for at least one year, usually around age forty-five to fifty. Once this occurs, a woman is no longer able to become pregnant.

Menses: Approximately monthly discharge of the unfertilized egg and the uterine lining as blood flows through the vagina.

Menstruation: Monthly cycle of hormone production and ovarian activities that prepares the body for pregnancy. If pregnancy does not occur, the uterine lining is shed, causing menses.

Miscarriage: Loss of a fetus.

Obesity: Abnormal excess of fat, usually defined as more than 20 percent over ideal body weight.

Oligomenorrhea: Light and infrequent menstrual flow.

Ovarian cyst: Noncancerous, fluid-filled sac located in or on the ovary that usually is a normal component of the ovulatory cycle.

Ovarian hyperstimulation: Rare complication that develops when the ovaries are overstimulated during the use of fertility medications such as clomiphene citrate or hMG. The ovaries enlarge and produce more follicles. This causes a buildup of fluid in the body, resulting in sudden weight gain, abdominal pain, nausea, and vomiting.

Ovaries: Two robin's egg–sized organs that produce the egg and female sex hormones.

Pituitary gland: Small gland within the brain that is responsible for regulating hormones associated with milk production and the menstrual cycle.

Placenta: Organ that develops within the uterus during pregnancy. It provides the fetus with nourishment, permits the elimination of waste products, and produces hormones needed to sustain pregnancy.

Progesterone: Hormone produced by the corpus luteum in the ovary, the adrenal glands, and the placenta (in pregnant women). It prepares the uterus for pregnancy and sustains the pregnancy.

Progestin: Name used for certain synthetic or natural progesterone agents. Usually contained in many types of birth control pills.

Prolactin: Hormone responsible for milk production.

Prostaglandins: Hormone-like proteins released by the uterine lining that cause uterine contractions, resulting in menstruation.

Proteins: Compounds that contain amino acids. Found in all living matter, proteins are essential for the growth and repair of animal tissue.

Provera: Medication prescribed to induce a period.

Puberty: Stage of human development between childhood and adulthood when secondary sex characteristics first become evident.

Steroids: Group of chemicals (considered hormones), many of which occur naturally in the body. Steroids can greatly affect bodily functions.

Testosterone: Male sex hormone responsible for the development of male characteristics.

Uterus: Organ in the pelvic region where the fertilized egg and fetus develop. Also called the womb.

Index

About the Authors

Angela Best Boss is the health education director of The Polycystic Ovarian Syndrome Association (PCOSA), the international PCOS support group. She also serves as director of communications for the local Indiana PCOS chapter. Her frequent articles on PCOS and infertility can be viewed at www.suite101.com and www.conceivingconcepts.com.

Ms. Best Boss has a bachelor's degree from Virginia Wesleyan College, Norfolk, Virginia, and a master's degree in counseling and ministry from Virginia Union University, Richmond, Virginia. She is also the author of two other books, *Surviving Your First Year As a Pastor: What Seminary Couldn't Teach You* (Judson Press, 1999) and *Heart of a Shepherd: Meditations for New Pastors* (Judson Press, 2000).

Ms. Best Boss lives in Indiana with her husband and children.

Evelina Weidman Sterling is a certified health education specialist and consultant to various nonprofit and government agencies in the area of evaluation and health services research. She previously worked for the American Association for Health Education, Health Resources and Services Administration, Gallaudet University, and the American Heart Association.

Ms. Weidman Sterling holds a bachelor of science degree in biology from Mary Washington College, Fredericksburg, Virginia, and a master's degree in health sciences from the Johns Hopkins University School of Hygiene and Public Health, Baltimore, Maryland. She lives in Atlanta, Georgia, with her husband and children.

Jerald S. Goldstein, M.D., is a reproductive endocrinologist and an OB/GYN physician in Dallas, Texas; he's on staff at Texas Health Presbyterian Hospital. He has extensive experience in infertility, polycystic ovarian syndrome, recurrent miscarriage, and third-party reproduction.

Dr. Goldstein is certified by the American Board of Obstetrics and Gynecology in both obstetrics and gynecology and reproductive endocrinology and infertility, a distinction held by fewer than 1,000 physicians in the country. He received his bachelor of science degree with honors from Tulane University, New Orleans, Louisiana, and graduated from the University of Texas Southwestern Medical School in 1992. He completed his residency at Oakwood Hospital, an affiliated hospital with the University of Michigan, and his fellowship in reproductive endocrinology and infertility at the University of Vermont.

Dr. Goldstein's past academic appointments include assistant professor, Department of Obstetrics and Gynecology, Division of Reproductive Endocrinology and Infertility, at the Washington University School of Medicine, St. Louis, Missouri. He has presented his research at the national meetings of the American Society of Reproductive Medicine and the Society of Gynecologic Investigation, and his research has been published in *Fertility and Sterility* and *Obstetrics and Gynecology.* He has lectured on a variety of topics related to reproduction and fertility and is a member of the American Society of Reproductive Medicine, American College of Obstetrics and Gynecology, as well as the Society for Reproductive Endocrinology and Infertility (SREI).

Dr. Goldstein and his wife, Jennifer, live in North Dallas, Texas, with their two sons, Ryan and Ben.

Dr. Goldstein may reached through his Web site: **fertilitydallas.com.**

Consumer Health Titles from Addicus Books

Visit our online catalog at www.AddicusBooks.com

Straight Talk about Breast Cancer—
   From Diagnosis to Recovery $15.95
The Stroke Recovery Book—
   A Guide for Patients and Families $14.95
The Surgery Handbook—
   A Guide to Understanding Your Operation $14.95
Understanding Lumpectomy—
   A Treatment Guide for Breast Cancer. $14.95
Understanding Parkinson's Disease—A Self-Help Guide . . . $19.95
Understanding Peyronie's Disease. $16.95
Understanding Your Living Will. $12.95
Your Complete Guide to Breast Augmentation
   & Body Contouring $21.95
Your Complete Guide to Breast Reduction & Breast Lifts . . $21.95
Your Complete Guide to Facelifts. $21.95
Your Complete Guide to Facial Cosmetic Surgery $19.95
Your Complete Guide to Nose Reshaping $21.95

To Order Books:

   Visit us online at: www.addicusbooks.com
   Call toll free: (800) 352-2873

For discounts on bulk purchases, call our Special Sales
Dept. at (402) 330-7493.